Chronic Disease Management

Chronic Disease Management

Chronic Disease Management

A Practical Guide

Edited by
Tessa Muncey and Alison Parker

palgrave

First published 2002 by
PALGRAVE
Houndmills, Basingstoke, Hampshire RG21 6XS and
175 Fifth Avenue, New York, N.Y. 10010
Companies and representatives throughout the world

PALGRAVE is the new global academic imprint of
St. Martin's Press LLC Scholarly and Reference Division and
Palgrave Publishers Ltd (formerly Macmillan Press Ltd).

ISBN 0–333–73693–1 paperback

This book is printed on paper suitable for recycling and
made from fully managed and sustained forest sources.

A catalogue record for this book is available
from the British Library.

10   9   8   7   6   5   4   3   2   1
11   10   09   08   07   06   05   04   03   02

Printed in Great Britain by Creative Print and Design (Wales), Ebbw Vale

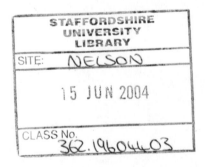

Contents

List of Boxes

List of Figures and Tables

Preface

Florence Nightingale's (1860) seminal text *Notes on Nursing* has the sub-title 'What it is and what it is not'. While in no way suggesting that this text emulates such a profound text on nursing, the sub-title provides a suitable description of the preface for this book; the editors feel it is important to stress what this book aims to do and what it does not.

The book sets out to give a practical guide to chronic disease management based on current evidence. It is not intended to provide a critical analysis of each concept, but where controversy occurs the reader will be directed to alternative sources. Within the book there are two styles of presentation. First, the tone and content of the general chapters are designed to make abstract concepts like assessment, team working and compliance accessible to practising nurses. Second, the practical chapters are written by practitioners who have used current theoretical knowledge underpinned by a wealth of experience to present chronic disease management in an accessible and practical format. Specialist nurses in fields such as asthma management who want to develop current practice with up to date knowledge may access the book, or the wider issues of chronic disease management may appeal to new practitioners.

The female gender has been used throughout the book to refer to the nurse. This is to reflect the larger numbers of nurses who are female but we hope it does not negate the expertise or experience of our male colleagues.

Acknowledgements

The editors and the publisher wish to thank the following for permission to use copyright material: The National Asthma and Respiratory Training Center, p. 90; Linda Pearce, p. 91; Martin Dunitz Ltd., p. 101a; Clement Clarke International Ltd., pp. 101–2; British Medical Journal, p. 103; Tayside Centre for General Practice, p. 72; Jenny Pool, pp. 105–6 and 125a–b; National Asthma Campaign, p. 122; British Journal of General Practice, p. 123; Glaxo Wellcome UK Ltd., p. 124; Churchill Livingstone, pp. 170–171; Professor Philip Ley, p. 219; Emap Healthcare Ltd., pp. 221, 223, 247–8.

While, every effort has been made to trace all the original copyright holders, if any have inadvertently been overlooked, the publisher will be pleased to make the necessary arrangement at the first opportunity.

List of Abbreviations

BTS   British Thoracic Society
WHO   World Health Organisation
BHS   British Hypertension Society
RCN   Royal College of Nursing

Notes on the Contributors

Joan Bendall is an independent nurse advisor in diabetes, Cambridge Diabetes Consultancy.

Shirley Crouch is a nurse teacher in curriculum development pre-registration at the Isle of Man Centre for Nurse Education.

Jan Davis is a nurse practitioner in Winchester.

Tessa Muncey is a principal lecturer at Homerton College, School of Health Studies, Cambridge.

Jenny Kelly is a senior lecturer at Homerton College, School of Health Studies, Cambridge.

Alison Parker is a part-time lecturer at Homerton College, School of Health Studies, Cambridge and a part-time practice nurse in Cambridgeshire.

Sue Paulson is a professional teaching associate at Homerton College, School of Health Studies, Cambridge and a part-time staff nurse in Palliative Care.

Janet Street is a practice nurse in Cambridge.

Sally Quilligan is a practice nurse in Cambridgeshire.

Part I

Self Care and Chronic Disease

1

Collaboration in Health Care?

TESSA MUNCEY

This chapter will examine the issues that nurses need to consider in order to contribute to a more successful collaboration in the future with patients and other healthcare practitioners and serve as a signpost to other chapters in the book. In a postmodern world of multiple realities, the idea of the one truth as promised in Newtonian physics has gradually given way to an idea of multiple truths, culminating in uncertainties as to how we can seek to improve the health of people in Western industrialised societies. Most recently, New Public Health recognizes the complex interactions between biological, social, environmental, and individual factors (Lupton, 1995). Instead of polarising explanations for ill health between extreme biological explanations and extreme social or lifestyle explanations it attempts to provide evidence that aims to understand the way these interactions work in society and within the individual. A core feature of this approach is to actively promote health in healthcare policies rather then focus on curative medicine.

Alongside these changes in health policy nursing has been slow to change. Nursing is traditionally connected with caring for the sick. Reinforcement of this link was made at the start of the National Health Service (NHS). The NHS came into being on 5 July 1948. It gave everyone the right to have his or her own doctor and to receive appropriate medical care free at the point of delivery. It grew out of a culture of widespread and accessible primary care dating back to the 1911 National Insurance Act. It gave rise to a professional tribalism, which led to competition between healthcare disciplines and a compliance model, which became unwieldy and ineffective (Davies, 1996; Soothill, Mackay and Webb, 1995). The financial burden of the NHS was thought to be both 'right and necessary both as a means of alleviating suffering and promoting a standard of health which is vital for the future well-being of the nation' (Houghton & Whittow, 1965, p. 11). Despite this dual emphasis on primary and secondary care, the power structures in the medical profession ensured that specialisation gave power through knowledge. Hospital specialists attracted the attention of politicians and commanded larger and larger portions of the budget to sustain increasingly sophisticated treatments supported by dramatic technological development. This led to secondary care and the diagnosis of sickness, rather than prevention, becoming the focus of healthcare. However, it was hoped that the subsequent improvement in the nation's health would place less pressure on a curative healthcare budget (NHS Act 1946 cited in Hill and Woodcock, 1949).

By the end of the 20th century, it was recognized that people's health and social needs were changing and the optimism of the originators of the NHS did not in fact materialise. Increased expectation of quality of life, expectations of quality of service and the enormous cost of healthcare provision led to tensions within the service. In its health strategy for England, *Saving Lives: Our Healthier Nation* (Department of Health, 1998b:1.17) the government set out its twin aims:

- to improve the health of the whole population by increasing the length of people's lives and the number of years people spend free from illness
- to improve the health of the worst off in society and to narrow the health gap.

As a result of these policy initiatives nurses are faced with the following challenges at the beginning of the 21st century:

- increasing elderly population
- provision of support in the community for chronic and life threatening diseases
- inequalities in health
- changes to trends in disease associated with obesity, mental illness and chronic non-communicable diseases
- changing technology.

The management of chronic disease embraces all these issues and has particular implications for all healthcare team members. However, developing alongside these changes in policy and practice was the notion of a public that wanted more say in their healthcare. The concept of 'informed consent' started to appear in the literature in 1972 despite having been discussed at the end of the Second World War. This reflects the growing trend of individuals wanting to be involved in decisions about their health care. Rather than compliance with the expert opinions of doctors and nurses, patients are demanding more say and partnership in healthcare choices.

To participate in a partnership patients need empowering, to make choices, rather than pressure to accept expert advice. This requires professionals who need skills of facilitation and teaching. Empowerment is a concept that can be seen extensively in research literature. Hokanson Hawks (1992, p. 609) defines it as 'the interpersonal process of providing the proper tools, resources and environment to build, develop and increase the ability and effectiveness of others to set and reach goals for individual and social ends'. In this state, an individual actually possesses a relatively high degree of power that enables them to make genuinely free choices.

User Groups

In embracing individualism, the western world has placed greater responsibility on individuals to take responsibility for their own health. The rise of mass consumer cultures has given ordinary people the chance to express their own preferences and their own identity. Knowledge is seen as highly relative, more democratic, local and individualised (Rosenau, 1992). Professionals, as guardians of the types of knowledge which are now being revalued, may feel threatened but will have to accept the inevitability of more equal partnerships with users. It has to be remembered that in community care users and carers do most of the work themselves. It is in the interests of efficient and effective service delivery to give them more say in how the services which supplement their input to self care and informal care are planned and allocated.

Understanding the incidence and prevalence of disease in local communities is vital in establishing healthcare priorities based on the real needs of the neighbourhood. Chapter 2 introduces the concept of epidemiology, which is a vital tool in establishing health-associated factors, and, more importantly, the functioning of the services related to health.

The Needs of the Individual with Chronic Disease

When diagnosed as having a chronic disease people have to grapple with the knowledge that very often there is no cure for their condition. For many their lives will be shortened and the quality reduced. If chronic disease is not to be considered a life sentence then attention has to be given to the needs of the person that will enable them to live a full and happy life within the constraints of their condition. (See Box 1.1.)

The process of nursing is a logical, systematic way of planning patient care. By making the process of nursing explicit, not just to colleagues but also to patients, it provides the key to empowering patients to take back

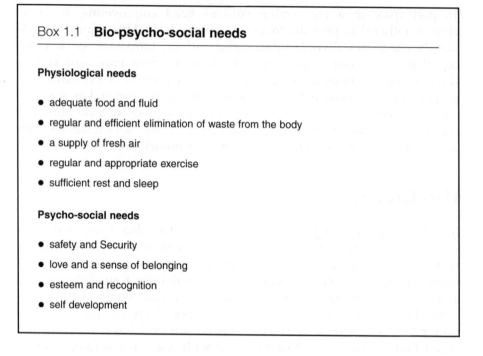

Box 1.1   **Bio-psycho-social needs**

Physiological needs

- adequate food and fluid
- regular and efficient elimination of waste from the body
- a supply of fresh air
- regular and appropriate exercise
- sufficient rest and sleep

Psycho-social needs

- safety and Security
- love and a sense of belonging
- esteem and recognition
- self development

responsibility for their own health. Plans of care must not prioritise the physiological needs at the expense of psycho-social ones. While the person may recognize their need for a balance of the physiological needs, in order to live a fulfilling life within the constraints of chronic disease, they also need to attend to the psycho-social needs. Proactive assessment is a key feature of the nursing contribution to the management of chronic disease. Chapter 3 outlines the principles of assessment and Chapters 4 and 5 relate this specifically to the assessment and management of asthma.

Role Boundaries

This shift from providers to service users has implications for the way health-care is organised. Much of the prevailing thoughts on the future of primary health care are that the multiplicity of groups involved in the delivery of care should be working more effectively together. This may result in 'co-operative decision making with team members each holding legitimate authority rather than on insular professional autonomy' (Bishop and Scudder, 1990). Brooking (1991) argues that the role boundaries between nursing and medicine are arbitrary and changing. She argues that a deliberate blurring of roles in multi-disciplinary clinical teams will lead to: collaboration in research; shared education and training; and partnerships between nurses and doctors in healthcare management. They will then be able to work together to develop new services based on the systematically identified needs of practice populations. In turn, this should lead to collaboration in providing an effective service and the use of both economic and clinical determinants of effectiveness.

The modernisation of the National Health Service to address this agenda started with the NHS (Primary Care) Act 1997. This allowed the establishment of more flexible personal medical services that could be more responsive to local needs and eventually led to the concept of Primary Care Groups. Primary Care Groups are groups of local healthcare and social care professionals who together with patient and Health Authority representatives take devolved responsibility for the healthcare needs of their local community. They are intended to bring GPs, nurses, and other local stakeholders together and give them a lead role in the planning, provision and development of local health services. In doing so, Primary Care Groups ensure that they pursue the development of the highest quality of provision for *all* patients within their area, while also acting to ensure the best value for money from the resources available to them. They have three main functions:

1. to improve the health of, and addressing health inequalities in, their communities;

2. to develop primary care and community services across the Primary Care Group;

3. to advise on, or commission directly, a range of hospital services for patients within their area which appropriately meets patients needs.

Primary Care Groups operate at one of four levels, and with the Health Act (Department of Health, 1999), repealing the law governing fundholding practices from 1 April 2000 groups operating at level three and four are known as Primary Care Trusts.

- *Level 1*: at a minimum, act in support of the Health Authority in commissioning care for its population, acting in an advisory capacity;

- *Level 2*: take devolved responsibility for managing the budget for health care in their area, acting as part of the Health Authority;

- *Level 3*: become established as freestanding bodies accountable to the Health Authority for commissioning care;

- *Level 4*: become established as free standing bodies accountable to the Health Authority for commissioning care, and with added responsibility for the provision of community services for their population.

To move forward primary healthcare initiatives are required to be sensitive to these new working arrangements, to allow the delegation of work to the health professional who can deliver it most cheaply, and to reflect the professional development of discrete groups, but above all to reflect the collaborative initiatives of a wide variety of healthcare providers and user groups. As over 95 per cent of the population are registered with a GP and on average consult a doctor four times a year (Williams, 1993), this means that the whole team should be well-placed to serve the needs of the users and to provide a tailor-made service by the most suitable, skilled, knowledgeable healthcare professional. The principles of team working are addressed in Chapter 6 followed by a team approach to the treatment and management of diabetes mellitus in Chapters 7 and 8.

Compliance or Empowerment?

While it could be argued that the advent of Primary Health Care Teams in 1974 paved the way for a team approach to patient care, in many ways they did little more than realign the attachment of nurses to GPs practices that existed in the 1960s. The historical approach to health care has been paternalistic. In trying to ensure the most cost effective treatment for the patient it was thought that at best too much information would confuse the patient and at worst would disempower the professional. It is recognized that most people are capable of making well-informed decisions about their health and lifestyle if they are given the right information, in an understandable form, at the right time.

However, if they decide not to comply with the recommendations of the healthcare professional it is also recognized that it is impossible to enforce compliance. For the professionals involved this requires having the confidence to develop a relationship with an individual, who sometimes may appear to have all the answers; who may have lived with their condition for long periods of time; or may be individuals who have ignored professional advice. Chapter 9 considers in detail the debates surrounding the nature of compliance and empowerment with Chapters 10 and 11 considering the importance of this in the treatment and management of people with hypertension.

Clinical Governance

Clinical governance sets out to do more than rename the associations between healthcare practitioners. It is about a shift in culture and attitude in the Health Service. In a few words, it is about putting doctors and nurses in charge of the way things are done and making both clinicians and managers accountable for the quality of patient care. The idea has emanated from the present governments proposal's to modernise the health service (NHS Executive, 1999).[1]

Clinical governance is a framework to help improve standards by making sure that organisations develop a culture, systems and ways of working which assure that quality of care is at the heart of the service. It includes clinical audit, risk management, evidence based practice, patient feedback, clinical supervision and continuing professional development and reflective practice. It requires true partnership between all clinicians: doctors, nurses, therapists and dieticians, and patients should be encouraged to have a say in decisions that affect them.

Changing Role and Qualities of the Nurse

To respond to these many changes in policy, resulting from a shifting demography, illness patterns and user group demands, the nurse's role has had to adapt and grow. Nurses working in the primary care setting have expanded considerably, particularly those working in General Practice. In 1993, practice nurses represented almost one-fifth of the estimated 50 000 whole-time equivalent nurses working in Primary Health Care (Hirst *et al.*, 1995) and this number has steadily increased. These nurses have a variety of role models, from the treatment room nurse to nurse practitioners (Stillwell and Bowling, 1996).

In order to help meet the needs of any person with healthcare deficits the nurse must be seen to have certain qualities. The good nurse can be seen to be guided as much by expertise as intuition (Benner, 1984). In a study examining the qualities of a good nurse, the ability to tolerate ambiguity and disengage from personal feelings, were found to be paramount (Muncey, 2000). Nurses who act as a rescuer, that is those who have the tendency to know what is right and impose a plan of care on the patient, will not facilitate the needs of the person with chronic disease.

The challenges of partnerships in chronic disease management are to recognize needs and create choices, acknowledge identity, allow dignity and create independence. These all require some elements of risk and some of the choices may not be the ones that the healthcare practitioner would choose. However, it is the patient who has to live with their choices and further experience of the disease may be required before they are able to come to terms with the adaptations which will alter their lives significantly. Within the auspices of clinical governance, the management of the person with chronic disease should be delegated to the most appropriate team member and this may often be the nurse. Protocols should clearly identify the roles of individual team members so that expertise can be developed appropriately. Nurses should be able to negotiate packages of care based on proactive nursing assessment using problem-solving skills that should enable the person to achieve a degree of normality within the constraints of the condition and have a good quality of life with minimal restrictions and minimal side effects. Chapter 12 considers the protocols that need to be in place in order to develop nurse-led clinics and Chapter 13 considers the depth of knowledge that would be required to facilitate the running of such a clinic for a person with epilepsy.

In the context of the changing nature of health care, this book considers the various aspects of the nurse's changing role and illustrates the knowledge skills and attitudes, which are required to fulfil them. With the devolvement of responsibility to nurse-led clinics, a more substantial level of knowledge is required within specialist areas. The organisation of nurses in the workplace has had to be more adaptable, which requires them to feel comfortable with change and the management of change. This has meant trying to overcome professional straitjackets where roles are clearly demarcated and rigid. Practices – which have existed unofficially, such as nurses prescribing treatments – are becoming formalised in nurse prescribing legislation. Chapter 14 considers the ethical and legal issues of such practices as nurse prescribing and responsibility for clinical updating that result from the changes outlined. This will enable the proactive nurse of the future to enter into negotiated packages of care with patients, where the emphasis is on offering choices rather than selecting preferred options and ultimately leaving the patient to carry out those healthcare practices which best fit their view of the risks that they face.

Conclusion

To rise to the challenge of improving the health of the whole population requires partnership between patients and healthcare practitioners. Empowered patients should be able to negotiate care packages that will minimise the long-term complications of chronic disease. Teams working under the auspices of clinical governance will maximise the best use of resources. The Primary Care Trusts will anticipate local health needs by using epidemiological principles and responding to evidence from research.

Note

1. See Appendix for website addresses offering comprehensive coverage of UK public sector information.

2

Epidemiology

JANET STREET

The word epidemiology is derived from the Greek and literally means 'studies upon people'. A comprehensive definition of epidemiology is described in Box 2.1. This broader definition recognizes that the modern study of epidemiology is concerned with the causes and occurrence of disease or conditions and, importantly the functioning of services related to health. With growing problems of limited resources and rationing, modern epidemiology is as much involved with the results of healthcare interventions as with known and potential risk factors, the latter commonly known as social, rather than the traditional medical, epidemiology. There is evidence that environment damages health (Draper, 1991). This was documented in two famous reports of the 1980s, *The Black Report* (DHSS, 1980) and *The Health Divide* (Whitehead, 1987). Commenting on these Townsend and Davidson (1992) highlighted the findings of inequalities in health, particularly in geographical distribution, accessibility to healthcare services, socio-economic deprivation and the resultant health problems. A Kings Fund project (Benzeval *et al.*, 1995) continues to highlight the persisting inequalities in health, no more so than in the area of socio-economic inequalities and health.

Nursing and Epidemiology

Epidemiology has traditionally been firmly placed with medicine within its medical model whereas nursing has been based around holism and

---

Box 2.1 **Definition**

'The study of the distribution and determinants of health-related states or events in specified populations and the application of this study to the control of health problems.' (Last, 1988)

---

naturalism. We are now in the age of planning, with health needs assessment, quality issues, the introduction of Primary Care Groups (PCGs) and Clinical Governance among the elements of NHS reforms outlined in *The New NHS, Modern, Dependable* (Department of Health, 1997) and *A First Class Service* (Department of Health, 1998). Whatever healthcare services are envisaged the fundamental issues of distribution, information, cost effectiveness and widespread health technology emerge, particularly so when seen against the 1990s background of cost reduction and rationing.

Epidemiology and Practice Nursing

Practice nursing has changed considerably in the past decade and this has been most apparent in the nurse's role in chronic disease management. To undertake their role practice nurses do not require knowledge of epidemiology but, if opportunities for disease prevention (primary, secondary or tertiary) and health promotion are to be taken, some knowledge of its application is required. Requirements for evidence based interventions must include:

- understanding the causes and risks of the disease or condition
- understanding the evidence and appraisal
- knowledge of the size, determinants and distribution of the disease
- understanding the principles of screening and its limitations for individuals and populations
- appreciation of the principles of prevention and health promotion
- knowledge of the importance of clinical audit
- evaluation of the services provided
- skills in personal reflection and ability to prioritise work personally and within the primary healthcare team and community/work setting.

Defining and Measuring Health

There are many different approaches to measuring health and the interpretations of the word 'health'. The lay and official account of health is multifactorial and changes over time and between different cultures and societies. It is probably easier to collect data on disease than on perceived ill health among the community, with the latter being more qualitative. This makes it difficult to undertake comparative studies.

Epidemiology focuses on disease and is criticized for not also including the positive and negative aspects of health. Attempts are being made to quantify the quality of health provision in areas of practice and community profiles.

Counts and Rates

Total numbers of cases of a condition or disease in a given population is one of the simplest measures in epidemiology. Whereas, a rate is a measure of how frequently an event happens. All rates are expressed as ratios, that is one number divided by another, the top figure being the numerator and the bottom the denominator. An example is where the numerator could be the number of flu cases in a population and the denominator the total population number

$$\frac{\text{Number of cases of flu (numerator)}}{\text{Number in the population (denominator)}}$$

This equation produces a fraction so we conventionally multiply crude rates by 100, 1000 or 10000 to produce a whole number. In the above example, by multiplying the crude rate by 100, it can be stated as 'so many cases of flu per 100 population', for example 3 per 100 or 3 per cent. The two most commonly used rates by epidemiologists are *prevalence rates* and *incidence rates*.

Prevalence and Incidence

These rates are used to measure the frequency of a disease or health condition in a given population.

Prevalence Rates

Prevalence rates measure the number of existing cases of a disease in a given population at a point in time or over a short period of time, such as a day.

$$\text{Prevalence} = \frac{\text{total number of exisiting cases of a disease at a point in time}}{\text{total population at a point in time}}$$

Incidence Rates

In comparison to prevalence rates, which are seen as a snapshot of the existing condition, incidence rates, describe the continuing occurrence of new cases of a disease over a period such as a year.

$$\text{Incidence} = \frac{\text{number of new cases in a given period}}{\text{population at risk in this period}}$$

Unlike prevalence, the denominator is not the total population, as not all the population is at risk. Expanding this, some of the population with chronic lifelong disease such as diabetes who, cannot develop it again, are removed from the population at risk – which is an important concept, as incidence refers to people who *could* become new cases.

Incidence rates are important when carrying out needs assessment or healthcare service planning, as they give a measure of the occurrence of new cases of a disease or a lifestyle habit such as smoking. This can be achieved by applying national rates to a given population over time. Changes in incidence rates show whether a particular disease is increasing or decreasing, which in turn alters the size of the 'population at risk'. It is sometimes difficult to interpret. If there is seen to be a decrease in a particular problem does this reflect the true success of a health promotion programme or is it the outcome of other factors?

Prevalence and incidence rates are not always 'clear cut' as there is an assumption made whether the individual or group has the disease or not. As we know in primary care, patients do not always fit into neat boxes. There are conditions, particularly in relation to chronic diseases such as hypertension, where the definition of diagnosis varies from practice to practice and so there is a variation of what constitutes hypertension. This is more problematic when looking at the extent of certain behaviours such as dietary habits, or what constitutes 'safe' alcohol consumption.

Identifying the amount of disease in the population is by data collection of mortality and incidence figures linked to morbidity.

Mortality

It has been a requirement since 1874 in the UK that births and deaths are registered. The system is organised by the Office of National Statistics (ONS). Cause of death is coded following an internationally agreed system, the International Classification of Disease (ICD). These ICD codes are also used for morbidity data. Statistics on cause of death are now *usually* based on the underlying disease. These statistics have problems between the main and underlying cause of death, as this may not be known at the time, but are generally considered to be complete. Information about death rates remains the most common source of information for health needs assessments, because they are easily available and reasonably reliable.

Morbidity

Morbidity data gives information about the extent of ill health. In comparison to mortality data, morbidity data gives knowledge of the full extent of ill health. However, morbidity data is notoriously difficult to collect, because the data is not available or not in a form that is easily collectable or meaningful. Information on morbidity mainly comes from health services activities. This has its problems, as it tends to alter as healthcare structures change and systems are updated, so rendering comparisons difficult. Current health service activity is in the form of consultation and treatment rates, which are recorded in activity analyses, hospital inpatient enquiries (HIE), cancer and infectious disease notification/registration and national studies of morbidity from general practice. This provides information about the extent of illness but not completely. As far as assessing the extent of illness in the community, not all ill persons are admitted to hospital and much illness is not seen by the GP but help is sought from friends and relatives, pharmacists or alternative therapists.

Market research is not carried out to determine the amount of ill health in the community, for example, analyzing 'over the counter' medication. Nevertheless, data available can give indications of the extent of ill health in different geographical areas and is used in planning health service provision. Much chronic illness and disability is not measurable, as the baseline data collected is relying on negative definitions of health and may fail to gather the full extent of morbidity. In measuring 'positive' health as well as 'negative' health it is important to take into account, the lay person's subjective measures of the interpretation of their own health. This important information in the form of *The General Household Survey* (GHS) is available from the ONS. A continuous survey running since 1971, it is based on a sample of the general population in private households in Great Britain. It records lay peoples' views about the nature and degree of severity of their own ill health or disability.

Research conducted by Bowling (1992) has questioned the importance of relying on negative definitions and measures of health such as mortality and morbidity data, as the latter does not tell us anything about the remaining 80 to 90 per cent of the population. Although it is difficult to measure positive health, Pickin and St Leger (1993) have concluded that the huge task of measuring areas such as social support and community involvement, it should be undertaken. They see the measures of social health and support as particularly important for nurses as being a positive contribution to the holistic approach.

Standardised Mortality Ratio (SMR)

When taking crude death rates and trying to make a comparison in different populations, it may be necessary to adjust the rate to take into account the age and sex profile of the populations being compared. Some parts of the population have a greater mortality rate than others, for example women have a lower mortality than men. Specific rates account for this by measuring the number of events occurring in a population sub-group, for example the mortality rate of females in social class 4 in different areas. The British population is classified according to occupation and within this classification social class 4 refers to those in a partly skilled occupation (OPCS, 1991). One such rate that takes into account these differences, is the SMR. The rate is calculated by using the number of 'expected' deaths and the actual number of deaths observed as such:

$$\text{SMR} = \frac{\text{observed number of deaths}}{\text{expected number of deaths}}$$

The figure is usually multiplied by 100. If the standard population and the population being compared had the same mortality experience, then the figure would be 100 because the expected and the observed number would be equal. If a population being compared has a figure greater than 100 then mortality in that population is higher than that in the standard; less than 100 means that the mortality is lower.

Cause, Risk, Prevention and Screening

As mentioned previously epidemiology is concerned with the distribution and determinants of disease. Simply, it is concerned with who gets ill, why they get ill and their treatment. This epidemiological information may contribute to understanding 'sickness' events and how they can be interpreted and prevented. The concepts of cause, risk or the probability of events and prevention are central to epidemiology. The concept of *risk* includes both the 'risk' that a person may develop a particular disease having been exposed to a potentially harmful agent and the 'risk' that a certain intervention will be affected by the outcome to the persons benefit or otherwise.

Risk Factors are different but not all are causal agents or determinants of the disease or condition. The notion that different exposures, behaviour and personal characteristics influence our risk of developing a disease or condition is not new. However the term 'risk factors' comes from modern epidemiology. Large cohort or prospective epidemiological studies (studies of people chosen before contracting the disease being studied) were started after the Second World War. One such study was carried out in the late 1940s in the small American town of Framlingham (Unwin *et al.*, 1997). Female residents aged 30 to 59 took part in medical examinations, health surveys and personal behaviour studies (now more commonly known as lifestyle checks) such as smoking and drinking habits. At the time, as in any cohort study, the participants were free of coronary heart disease (CHD) and were re-examined several times over many years to look at the incidence of CHD. Increased risk of developing heart disease was associated with smoking, hypertension and high serum cholesterol levels, amongst others. These were the basis of many studies that determined the risk factors for heart disease today.

Cause

Few diseases have a single 'cause'. Most are the result of susceptible individuals being exposed to more than one causative agent. There are many factors that may influence disease development in addition to direct cause; an example is the influenza virus. It can be a complex situation relating cause to disease as chance could play its part. The observation that a disease is statistically associated with a suspected agent does not always mean it is the cause. The incidence of lung cancer in heavy smokers is around 20 times higher than in non-smokers. This relative risk indicates a strong association between cigarette smoking and lung cancer. It would be very difficult to say that cigarette smoking causes lung cancer. One cannot reach this conclusion without taking into consideration two questions:

- first, was the association found between exposure and the outcome in a study real? We need to know more about the study and reliability of evidence.

- second, association does not always mean causation. Assessing whether an association is likely involves epidemiology, but also needs to include evidence from other disciplines such as psychologists, economists, sociologists and so on.

An example of the latter is evidence that diabetes is on the increase in the UK and other parts of the world. There is a known association between diabetes in the population and measures of wealth such as gross national product (GNP). Perhaps the increase is linked to dietary changes such as increased sugar in our daily diet. This change in its turn is related to, for example, complex farming subsidies. So, reducing the prevalence of diabetes in the community requires a broad policy management change. Most chronic diseases have multiple causes, and particular causative factors or agents may cause more than one disease. MacMahon and Pugh (1970) have described this complexity, as the 'web of causation'. Practice nurses need to be aware of these broader causative agents.

Risk

According to the dictionary risk is 'hazard, chance of bad consequences' (Garmonsway, 1969). In epidemiology, according to Fletcher *et al.* (1988), it is also about the chance or probability of events occurring. Risk refers to the likelihood that 'people who are without disease, but are exposed to certain factors (risk factors), will acquire the disease'. Unlike the dictionary definition the event need not be undesirable. Concepts of risk, or probability of events, are central to the science of epidemiology.

Figure 2.1 gives a picture of the complexity of causation with an emphasis on the biological or genetic aspects of clinical epidemiology, whereas the emphasis in social epidemiology lies on sociological and political factors. This flowchart is applicable to causes of disease but can also be applied to individual health and the different components that play a part.

Absolute Risk

This is the same as incidence for the whole population.

Figure 2.1   Causal links in clinical epidemiology

Socio/cultural/political
factors

↓

Personal   →   Individuals health or   →   Future
Lifestyle   disease   outcomes
Health beliefs   consequences

↑

Biological or genetic
causes

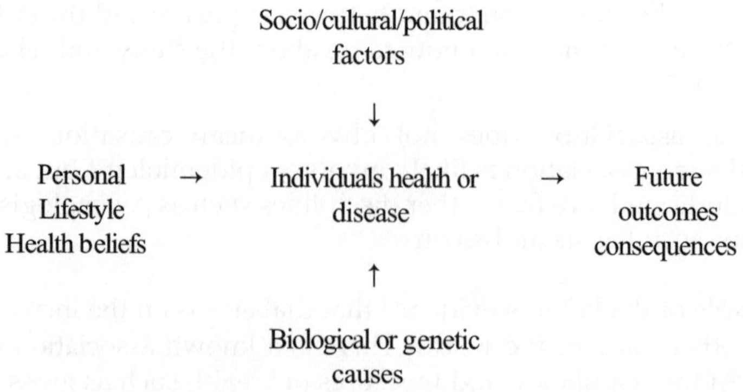

Relative Risk

Used to compare the incidence of a disease or condition in a group with a particular attribute or exposure to a group without. The relative risk score is:

Incidence in the group with attribute or exposure
Incidence in group without attribute or exposure

An example taken from a study in 1951 of British doctors and their smoking habits shows a strong association between mortality from lung cancer and smoking (relative risk of 17.1) (Unwin *et al.*, 1997). An exposure that is positively associated with the occurrence of a disease is called a risk factor for that disease for example smoking and lung cancer.

Attributable Risk

Used to provide an assessment of how much a disease could be seen to be due to exposure and so how it *might* be prevented if the exposure is removed.

Relative and attributable risk provides two very different types of health information. The latter has a more useful and meaningful concept in clinical practice since it indicates the probability of disease in those who are exposed. It is useful to advise preventive health measures aimed at the population. Information about risk factors may be useful in a variety of ways:

- *PREDICT* future disease incidence
- *DIAGNOSIS* for example a rash in a pregnant woman who is known to have rubella antibodies eliminates one disease – a case of the absence of the risk factor
- *PREVENTION* of disease by the removal of the risk.

It is necessary for the nurse to know the relative and attributable risk associated with exposure to certain activities such as smoking, alcohol consumption, non-compliance to medication and so on.

Prevention

Prevention has been classified at three levels: primary, secondary and tertiary (see Box 2.2). In each of these, it is essential to know the life history of the disease.

Box 2.2 **Definition of levels of prevention**

- Primary prevention relates to activities that attempt to stop harmful effects from occurring, for example vaccination of children.

- Secondary prevention aims at detection of disease in its early stages when treatment can be used to stop the condition from progressing, for example hypertension screening and intervention, and determining risk factors in a patient at risk of developing heart disease.

- Tertiary prevention covers the areas of activity where the disease is known but measures are taken to prevent further deterioration or in some cases death; an example is organ transplant.

Natural History of the Disease

Following causality, the second most important concept underpinning epidemiology is understanding the natural history of disease. Studying how the disease occurs and its progression is important in knowing when an intervention should take place in the form of screening or treatment. Fletcher *et al.* (1998) define the natural history of a disease 'as the way in which the condition develops without any medical intervention'. This is important in distinguishing it from medical intervention, and is then described as the clinical course of a disease.

In many conditions it is difficult to ascertain accurately the natural cause of the disease. This can be due to peoples' accounts of how they see a certain condition progressing and how they view it as part of their life. In many chronic diseases it is unlikely that accurate or reliable accounts of progress can be established. Prognosis is an important part of the process as it gives a forecast of future events to be used in the management of care given and for the patient to have some idea of progression. In screening, it is important to identify at what point the disease can be detected and when intervention is likely to be effective. An example of a screening procedure where the progression of a disease is not totally understood is in cervical cancer. It is recognized that there are stages in the disease developing from mild to moderate, to severe dysplasia that is seen as an early stage of cervical cancer.

Health Promotion

Health promotion includes both health education and preventative measures aimed at early detection of disease or disability. There are a range of activities aimed at promoting the good health of client groups. Health promotion has become a large part of the practice nurse workload (Department of Health, 1997) particularly since the introduction of *The New GP Contract* (Department of Health, 1990). This reflected changes in health care in the 1980s, with a greater emphasis placed on primary rather than secondary care. Many factors brought this about, the biggest being that in terms of cost, prevention is cheaper than cure. Another factor was Britain's membership of the World Health Organisation (WHO) and the commitment of member countries to 'health for all by the year 2000'. The end of the 1980s saw the publication of many social policy documents, with the government emphasizing the importance of health promotion and the prevention of ill health and, ultimately, the importance of reducing the high rates of mortality and morbidity from preventable diseases. These Green and White papers included *Promoting Better Health* (DOH, 1988), *Working with Patients* (DOH, 1989b), and *The Health of the Nation: Strategy for Action* (DOH, 1992).

With practice nurses developing an increasing role within primary care this area of work will continue to expand. This was highlighted for example in a study carried out in Oxford (Fullard *et al.*, 1987) where they concluded that 'ascertaining the major risk factors for cardiovascular disease in primary care may be substantially improved by an opportunistic, systematic approach using practice nurses'. The introduction of specific clinics in General Practice enables practice nurses to play an important role in disease prevention. Campbell *et al.* (1998) looked at the effects of secondary prevention clinics run by practice nurses on the health of patients with CHD. The study showed that 'within their first year secondary prevention clinics improved patient's health and reduced hospital admission'. Practice nurses in their contact with patients, not necessarily ill, are able to carry out opportunistic health promotion and screening.

However, Ross *et al.* (1994) showed that although the majority of practice nurses were willing to develop participation in health promotion, the lack of formal training meant that a large number of nurses were not prepared for the broad range of tasks required to be undertaken.

Screening

The definition of screening is 'The presumptive identification of unrecognised disease or defect by the application of tests, examinations or other procedures which can be applied rapidly. Screening tests sort out the apparently well persons who probably have a disease from those who probably do not.' (Last, 1988:118). Screening is about looking for health problems, but if not planned and delivered correctly, it can be ineffective, inappropriate and an unethical attempt at preventive health care.

Is Screening Worthwhile?

1. Earlier detection of a disease or known risk factors for disease or disability may lead to more effective intervention and a better prognosis for the patient.

2. Early detection of disease benefits both the individual and society, if the carrier of the disease is a hazard to others, for example screening for certain blood borne diseases among blood donors with Hepatitis B and C, HIV and so on.

The Principles of Screening

Devised by Wilson and Jungner (1968) for the WHO in the 1960s the ten Principles of screening (see Box 2.3) are still used as a basis to assess the viability of screening tests. These are quality assurance issues based around the disease, the test, follow up and treatment and the economic costs.

Box 2.3 **Principles for screening**

1. The condition sought should pose an important health problem.
2. The natural history of the disease should be well understood.
3. There should be a recognizable early stage.
4. Treatment of the disease at an early stage should be of more benefit than treatment started at a later stage.
5. There should be a suitable test.
6. The test should be acceptable to the population.
7. There should be adequate facilities for the diagnosis and treatment of abnormalities detected.
8. Screening should be repeated determined by the natural history of disease.
9. The chance of physical and psychological harm to those should be less than the chance of benefit. The cost of screening should be balanced against the benefit it provides.

Source: Wilson and Jungner (1968).

The Disease

The condition sought should pose an important health problem. In addition, the natural history of the disease should be understood. There would be no support for setting up a screening programme for diseases not considered important health problems. It does not need to be regarded as a major problem, as some rare diseases can be effectively screened and be cost effective for example phenylketonuria in the new-born. The disease must be an important problem having a direct effect on the length or quality of life. An example is the mass x-ray-screening programmes that were introduced in the 1940s when tuberculosis was a major threat. This screening programme was withdrawn in the 1980s once the threat had diminished.

There should be a recognizable early stage. Progression from the early or recognized latent stage must be understood. Identification of pre-invasive states by screening may then go on to be of considerable benefit to the patient by reducing the incidence of invasive cancer and subsequent mortality. Decisions to implement breast-screening programmes were only possible once detection of the disease at a pre-clinical stage was identified (Forrest, 1986).

Treatment of the disease at an early stage should be of more benefit than treatment at a later stage. In a climate of cost-effectiveness this is important, as early intervention may reduce the costs of treatment at a later stage. The treatment of congenital hypothyroidism is an example of this.

There should be a suitable test to identify those at risk. Screening methods should detect a high proportion of asymptomatic disease at stages where prognoses can be improved by early detection. There is a potential for developing new screening techniques informed by an increased identification of risk factors, particularly in the area of genetics. The test itself should have certain criteria applied, see Box 2.4. The sensitivity of a test is indicated by the ability to detect a disease and the specificity of a test is the ability to exclude people who do not have the disease.

The test should be acceptable to the population at risk. Acceptability by the individual to attend a screening programme is a very personal thing and can be influenced by many factors (see Box 2.5). Education about the screening programme is vital in order to encourage an individual to attend.

Follow-up and Treatment

There should be adequate facilities for the diagnosis and treatment of abnormalities detected. It is important in screening that there are adequate facilities

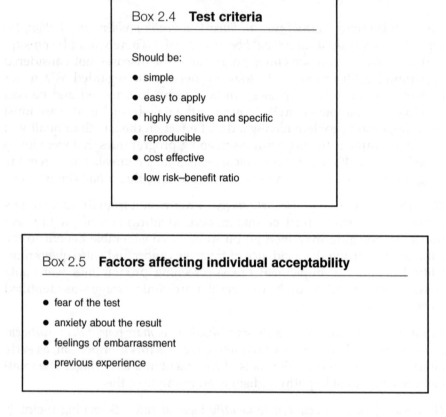

Box 2.4 **Test criteria**

Should be:

- simple
- easy to apply
- highly sensitive and specific
- reproducible
- cost effective
- low risk–benefit ratio

Box 2.5 **Factors affecting individual acceptability**

- fear of the test
- anxiety about the result
- feelings of embarrassment
- previous experience

for diagnosis and treatment as high levels of anxiety are created by positive results.

Screening should be repeated as determined by the natural history of the disease. Recall procedures must be effective and available. Knowledge of the natural history of the disease determines the intervals between routine screenings.

The chance of physical or psychological harm to those being screened should be less than the chance of benefit. It is important that health professionals are aware of the advantages and disadvantages of screening both physical and psychological. Informed choice by the individual is paramount when accepting a screening procedure.

Economic Costs

The cost of screening should be balanced against the benefit it provides. The cost of contacting and informing the population, carrying out the tests and any subsequent treatment must be economically balanced against the benefits.

Effectiveness Analysis

There are criteria to be considered when evaluating the effectiveness of screening programmes. Costs and benefits might be personal or social as well as economic and must include:

- the test must be acceptable to both target group and screener. It should be quick, simple, non-invasive and hazard free.

- the test must be reproducible. When applied by the same or different observers at different times, the test should give similar results. This begs the question 'are the screeners being screened'?

- the test must have being validity, giving the ability to separate individuals who have the disease from those who have not.

The Ethics of Screening

The ethical nature of the screening test is an important issue to consider, as part of a national programme within the surgery. The health practitioner is accountable for the outcome of screening so when a patient is invited or opportunistically offered screening the test must meet the basic criteria of efficacy and there must be facilities for follow up. There is also the question of media or public demand for a national screening test that is not yet specifically sensitive for example blood testing for prostate cancer in asymptomatic men (Gerard and Frank-Stromburg, 1998). The effects of raising anxiety levels in patients must be considered when carrying out screening tests, especially if the treatment or change in lifestyle involved is against their health beliefs.

Requirement for a Successful Screening Service

Other than fulfilment of the set criteria there are many factors that influence the success of a screening programme (see Box 2.6).

Why Does a Screening Programme Fail?

Not all screening programmes are successful and the reasons for this are outlined in Box 2.7.

Box 2.6   **Successful screening requirements**

- Adequate resources are available for undertaking screening, examining the individual and finally reporting back the results.
- Managerial skills and protocols are in place for making and keeping appointments for screening and chasing up non-attenders.
- Acceptability of the screening arrangements by the population.
- Ability to target the population and have call and recall lists that are up to date.
- Maintaining adequate coverage of target groups.
- Informing the client population adequately.
- Ongoing monitoring by audit of the efficiency and effectiveness of the screening programme both locally and nationally.

Box 2.7   **Reasons for screening failure**

- Target population is not reached.
- Tests are not sufficiently sensitive or specific.
- Treatment is not implemented following detection.
- The natural course of the disease is not changed by treatment.
- Inconsistency of screeners due to lack of training, incompetence or negligence.

Screening and the Practice Nurse

Increasing demand on health promotion and screening activities in primary care, mostly since the changes in the GP contract from 1990, has seen the delegation of this work to practice nurses who can participate in the screening of the population in several ways (see Box 2.8). The term screening is often applied to the over 75 check but is inappropriate as it is essentially a health check.

Mass Screening

Includes national screening programmes for breast and cervical cancer, whereby the practice nurse may undertake the smear test and give advice

---

Box 2.8 **Practice nurses role in screening**

- Inviting the individuals for screening and motivating them to attend without raising anxiety levels.
- Counselling about screening: outlining the benefits and limitations thereby empowering the individual to make an informed decision.
- Giving health education.
- Communicating results with an informed approach and being able to answer any questions.
- Advising on choices available following a positive result: for example in a case of raised cholesterol.
- Helping individuals to make necessary lifestyle changes.

---

to women on breast disease. Patients attend on an individual and voluntary basis.

Routine Screening

Antenatal screening is one example of practice nurse involvement within the Primary Health Care Team (PHCT). The registration health check could be seen as a screening activity, seeing all new patients registering with a practice between the ages of 5 and 75.

Opportunistic Screening

An example of opportunistic screening would be checking the rubella status of a woman currently using contraception but who is planning a family in the near future.

Selective Screening

Can be directed towards high-risk groups, for example:

- checking the blood pressure levels of diabetic patients
- screening for other CHD risk factors in a newly diagnosed hypertensive

On an individual basis the practice nurse has a large role within any screening programme.

Evaluation and Audit

When a member of the PHCT is involved in setting up any form of care for their practice population, some form of evaluation should be built in. Quality assurance of care being given is paramount, in the climate of cost effectiveness and efficiency of service. Professional organisations such as the Royal College of Nursing (RCN) and the Royal College of General Practitioners (RCGP) working with the Department of Health (DOH) and independent policy centres have played a crucial part in the policy agenda for assuring quality.

As a practice nurse quality assurance involves being aware of both one's own and one's colleagues values in the standards of care. It is important that when assessing and auditing any activity within the practice there must be a previously defined desired standard of care. When setting standards, assessing and auditing are two separate issues. When a desired standard has been planned, the nurse should ensure that it is achievable, observable, desirable and measurable within the Code of Professional Conduct (UKCC, 1992) and by constantly reassessing the quality of work, the practice nurse can help ensure that the standards are maintained. Audit is useful in assessing where the practice is at a point in time and to help introduce change. The concept of quality assurance lies in the practice nurse being aware of the roles and standards expected.

Research

The Briggs Report (1972) pointed the way for the need for nursing to base its practice on research, rather than traditional and sometimes ritualistic methods. The importance of basing nursing practice on quality research has been highlighted in many documents and government directives since the Briggs Report (Department of Health 1989a, 1993). Research-based practice is seen as the channel for forming the basis for delivery of effective and efficient nursing care and as a standard in the professionalism of nursing. In the field of evidence-based medicine, the nurse's role in research has been to assist in data collection. They have also contributed to health care by implementing procedures based on the results of research. More recently, nurses have become interested in the effects of screening, particularly on women. Foster (1995, p.128) suggests that 'cancer screening provides a whole range of benefits to all those involved in providing them.

There is as yet no conclusive proof that these programmes provide enough benefits to those women pulled into them to outweigh their well documented physical and emotional costs'. Screening for lung cancer in the 1960s was abandoned in favour of primary prevention. Nurses may become involved in research into the primary prevention of other potentially fatal diseases such as breast cancer. Secondary prevention fits the medical model of health where it is marketable and profitable particularly in 'fee for service' medical systems. Nurses, with their interest in holistic care, are well placed to ask questions about the effects of lifestyle on ill health that may highlight factors leading to primary prevention.

Conclusion

In establishing the causes and occurrence of disease, as well as studying the functioning of services related to health problems, decisions about limited resources and rationing of health care can be made appropriately. Identification of risk factors is a key feature of modern epidemiology and underpins healthcare practices such as screening and primary prevention.

Part II

Assessment of Chronic Disease

3

Assessment

TESSA MUNCEY

Information becomes education only when it is given in the context of the patients life (Brown 1997)

Early in my district-nursing career, I had a salutary lesson in the meaning of disease to a patient that was in distinct contrast to the prevailing medical model of the health service. A lady in her eighties with chronic venous ulceration to her legs under went a radical programme of management of her leg ulcer, which resulted for the first time in many years in the ulcerated areas becoming healed. As a new and keen district nurse I was very pleased with the progress and was puzzled by the patients increasing anxiety as the ulcer healed. Anticipating that her anxiety was related to the proposed end of the nurse's visit, I reassured her that occasional visits would be necessary to reassess the condition of her legs following recovery and also that she could be named as someone who might benefit from a regular visit from a local sixth former. Nothing would placate her and in exasperation one day I asked her what she was so worried about. She very sadly told me that for years she had seen a regular discharge from her leg, which she had decided was her body's way of rejecting 'the badness' from her body. If it was now healed, she was very concerned that this same 'badness' would continue to circulate around her body and cause a problem somewhere else. In assuming that we shared a common view of the physiology of the body, albeit fairly limited on her part, I had failed to ask the relevant questions that went to the heart of the problem.

This story is analogous with much of the failure of nursing assessment. If assumptions about disease and the meaning of ill health are not explored with the patient then any resulting plan will be doomed to failure. Any plan of care that does not have meaning to the patient will result in non-compliance and a waste of the scarce resources.

The misperceptions about the nature of nursing are understandable if they are only viewed as carrying out a series of psychomotor skills. What is more difficult to see is the affective and cognitive domain that is also

33

inherent in their actions. It is easy to observe a nurse carrying out a bed bath but it is almost impossible to see the other dimensions of this skill. The consideration of cultural requirements in respect of that patient and the evidence about pressure area development that may indicate special attention to various areas of the body. Positive body image is an important factor to a patient's quality of life achieved, by attending to personal requirements. As the nurse conducts the task consideration is given to privacy, psychological safety and the opportunity taken for health teaching. It is paradoxical that nurses appear to receive the greatest recognition from the patient who recovers from a range of side effects to their condition. The skilled proactive nurse who, by accurate assessment prevents the side effects occurring, may be in danger of going unnoticed because the patient is not aware of what could have happened without knowledgeable interventions.

Making the process of nursing explicit, not just to colleagues but also to patients, is the key to empowering patients to take back responsibility for their own health. By agreeing a basic philosophy within a team, recipients and providers of care should avoid a chaotic and uncoordinated delivery. The process of nursing is a logical, systematic way of planning the care a patient needs, but it still needs a framework within which to operate. Since the late 1970's assessment has been known to the nurse as the first part of the nursing process. At worse it is misconstrued as the collection of biographical data and physiological observations from the patient, at best it is confused with the practical experience of documentation of the data and often confused with the identification of problems without reference to the wider lifestyle issues that confront all patients. Assessment by the expert nurse is almost invisible. It is a cognitive process that to the observer can only be identified in the representation that is made in the nursing notes as a resumé of the process. The end result of assessment is the identification of actual and potential problems but these can only be arrived at after a detailed and systematic review of the whole person.

Almost anyone can be a nurse. Caring relatives, friends and neighbours carry out complex nursing care. Individuals can learn the intricacies of caring for even the most sick and disabled person. Mothers learn to balance the diet and medication of the young diabetic and juggle the lifestyle and inhalers of the energetic young asthmatic. Partners cope with rehabilitation following stroke and oversee the journey through the ravages of illness from cancer. What these 'nurses' learn to do is react to problems that arise or follow instructions from a qualified practitioner. They may acquire the necessary knowledge that enables them to cope with this one condition. This reactive approach to care may lead to unforeseen problems occurring or side effects developing that could have been prevented.

The professional nurse should be proactive, that is an attempt to anticipate problems before they arise. This approach is based on a wide body of knowledge and the ability to carry out a multifaceted approach to assessment of the patient and their environment.

Nursing History

The main purpose of the doctor in health care is to diagnose illness and prescribe treatment. This leaves the nurse with responsibility of helping the patient to understand the meaning of the condition and negotiate a plan of care with them, which takes account of complex lifestyle issues.

The majority of nurses work in teams and rely on carefully constructed communication to ensure continuity of care within patient care and between patient care. Without some systematic approach to both assessment and planning of care the implementation may well be chaotic and uncoordinated (see Box 3.1). The purpose of taking a nursing history is to collect information with which to identify the patients needs and problems (see Box 3.2). This information will then provide feedback to inform the deliberations of the wider healthcare team and provide the focus for negotiating a care plan with the patient. During the process of assessment, a variety of measurements will be taken. These may be objective measures such as physiological readings or subjective measures such as observation of non-verbal behaviour. The final stage of the assessment process is to review the information that has been collected and distil from it the actual and potential problems that need to be addressed. In the management of chronic disease it is vital that this last process be completed with the complete co-operation of the patient, otherwise non-compliance in the longer term can be almost guaranteed.

Assessment not only needs to establish the normal life pattern of the individual but to ascertain how important particular aspects are. If a person has an occupation that necessitates them entertaining clients at lunchtime a great deal, and the care plan requires some attention to their

---

Box 3.1 **What is assessment?**

- A means of measurement.
- Collection of information.
- Reviewing information.
- Identification of needs and problems.

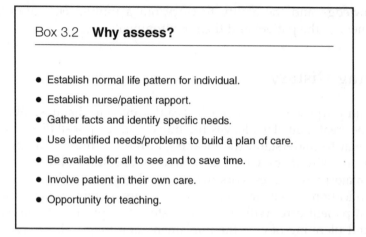

Box 3.2 **Why assess?**

- Establish normal life pattern for individual.
- Establish nurse/patient rapport.
- Gather facts and identify specific needs.
- Use identified needs/problems to build a plan of care.
- Be available for all to see and to save time.
- Involve patient in their own care.
- Opportunity for teaching.

diet, then it is necessary to consider ways that this might be achieved without suggesting that dining out will be a problem. If a young asthmatic is very keen on sport then the management of the disease must include advice and interventions that allow sporting activity to take place. If the best advice for the patient is to give up a particular lifestyle then they must have sufficient detail on which to decide whether to follow the advice. If a cat loving person with asthma is found to be allergic to cat fur then they may decide that on balance they would rather live with the consequences of owning the cat than to be asymptomatic without it. It is important that the person understands the rationale behind the advice and for the nurse to accept that the patient may have a different set of priorities.

Assessing patients in their own home provides a much richer source of assessment information. The nurse can use all her senses to establish the lifestyle of the individual and their family. It will be possible to soak up the sights, sounds and smells of an individual's life to use as the basis for discussion. Knowledge of local conditions, policies and facilities will greatly enhance this process. The house and its physical environs are immediately to view, but the assessor will still need information about any local environmental issues that may detract from compliance with a healthcare plan. For example regular attendance at a clinic for check-ups will be dependent on that person's ability to get to the centre. If they are not a driver or do not have regular access to a car then an affordable and accessible public transport system is required. In consideration of an individual's eating habits it will be possible to ascertain the conditions they have for the preparation and cooking of the meal as well as the pressing considerations of other family members and the convenience or otherwise of shopping facilities.

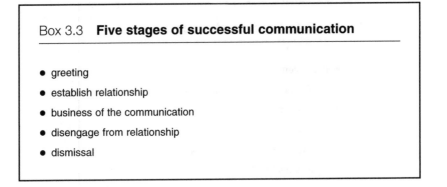

Box 3.3 **Five stages of successful communication**

- greeting
- establish relationship
- business of the communication
- disengage from relationship
- dismissal

If the person is being assessed in a clinic or ward then this information will have to be ascertained by careful questioning. A vital aspect in this discussion will be the setting-up of a good rapport with the person; successful communication depends on the establishment of the relationship (see Box 3.3). This relationship may well develop over a period of time but almost certainly the first meeting will set the scene for the others that follow. The greeting should always be warm, friendly and address the person by name with a smile if possible. Establishing a relationship may be to enquire after the family, briefly comment on an item of news or the weather during which time the person can make him or herself comfortable. During this brief encounter, it will be possible to establish their level of hearing and levels of anxiety. As they walk towards you in greeting, it is a ready-made assessment of their mobility.

Although the patient is a key person in the assessment process, other sources of information should be utilised particularly if the patient is very ill or unable to provide a full description of their needs due to physical disability. There are four other main sources of assessment (see Box 3.4). Family and friends will be an important source of information, particularly to assess their potential support in the patient's future plan of care. In the team approach to health care patients may choose to reveal different pieces of information to different members of staff, so a comprehensive assessment will include the information disclosed to nursing colleagues and other healthcare staff. Medical records will provide a detailed background of previous healthcare problems, but may be limited on the patient's reaction to the treatments offered, whereas the information provided by relatives and friends may give a more accurate picture of how the patients feels without in-depth knowledge of the medical interventions. The nursing records should bridge the gap between the two. The other two aspects of assessment require the collection of subjective and objective data. Observation requires a detailed description of what the nurse sees together with accurate measurements of physiological states.

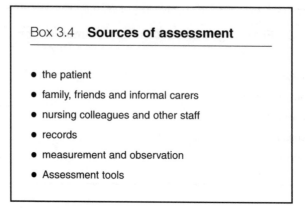

Box 3.4 **Sources of assessment**

- the patient
- family, friends and informal carers
- nursing colleagues and other staff
- records
- measurement and observation
- Assessment tools

Assessment of Eating Habits

The five sources of information will now be used to demonstrate how a patient's dietary needs and preferences can be assessed. *The patient* could tell you what they like to eat when they are well and when they are sick. Many people carry the behaviours of childhood illness into their adult lives. Eating when ill may vary from always eating something that is good for you to treating oneself to something special despite its poor nutritional content. *The patient* can explain the pattern of meals in a day: that is, how many meals a day they eat and at what times; how their diet changes through the seasons and for special occasions such as Christmas. They will be able to describe any cultural preferences. This may be indicated by ethical or religious responses such as vegetarianism or the need for halal or kosher preparation. Their personal selection of certain foods depends on their beliefs about the value of certain foods together with their availability and past experience. They will be able to describe their knowledge of nutritional values of certain foods and how they prepare and cook it. They will know how much they have to spend on food and whether the shops are easily accessible. They might give you an accurate assessment of their weight and alcohol intake, but these are areas that are notoriously sensitive and might be underestimated.

The patient will be able to indicate whether their mouth is comfortable when they eat, whether they have all their own teeth or dentures and whether any foods upset them in any way. They may also be aware of the dietary needs of any medication they take such as drugs that should be taken with or after food, or drugs like mono oxidase amino inhibitors for depression, where certain foods should be avoided.

Family, friends and informal carers will provide supporting evidence for the facts that the patient furnishes. They may indicate the extent to which they are prepared to accommodate any changes to diet that may need to be incorporated into a plan of care. They may express a willingness to take on some of the responsibility for providing food such as shopping or cooking if the patient has a deficit in these areas. The nurse will also gain an awareness of the extent to which the patient's eating habits are affected by the needs of the rest of the family.

Health care colleagues will provide evidence that supports or negates the patient's story. In the initial assessment, they may have been *anxious* to give an ideal version of their eating habits rather than an accurate depiction. This might be for a variety of reasons such as giving the information they think is required, being embarrassed by what they do or because they have forgotten certain information. The wider the view the more accurate the picture and in their association with the patient other colleagues may collect pieces of the jigsaw which give a more detailed picture. This picture might include insight into whether the patient eats to live or lives to eat and even an assessment of the depth and breadth of knowledge that a patient might have of the nutritional content of food.

Previous nursing and medical records will indicate anything that changes the digestive process. Any malfunctioning system in the body may have implications for eating and drinking: changes to the endocrine system may result in the need for a dietary regime that controls the regulation of blood sugar; the circulatory system may require a diet that reduces cholesterol; an impaired renal system may require a low protein diet. While the digestive system itself has a myriad of places that could be problematic, there may be teeth missing or ill-fitting dentures that result in chewing difficulties. The patient may have a history of constipation and gastric upsets may well indicate allergies or intolerance to certain foods.

Measurements and observations that the healthcare team might make are the patient's weight and height giving a Body Mass Index. Cholesterol levels might be monitored to indicate the potential for future or current cardiovascular disease. Blood glucose might be measured in order to detect diabetes or to monitor its treatment. Looking at the patient may give a good overview of the patient's dietary status: the texture and quality of skin will indicate the adequacy of nourishment and hydration. If the clothes the patient is wearing are tight or very loose fitting careful investigation may indicate a gain or a loss in weight recently. If the patient is observed in situations where they are eating or are able to cook, the effect of mobility, dexterity and the ability to handle cooking utensils can be observed.

Assessment tools have materialised to streamline the acquisition of information and assess the risk factors inherent in certain areas. It could be argued that to the knowledgeable, experienced nurse these tools are a useful checklist to enable them to arrive at a carefully considered insight into the needs of the patient. In the inexperienced hands, they are just a checklist which can be scored without an in-depth consideration of the wider issues. A checklist for dietary assessment will prove ineffective, unless all of the factors described above are taken into consideration, together with research evidence from dietetics and a consideration of the meaning of food in a patient's life.

Models of Nursing

Assessment requires a framework in which to work. A framework, which reflects the philosophy of health care, which fits the particular environment and client group, and resources available. In nursing these may take the form of a variety of nursing models. Nursing has developed alongside the medical model that incorporates a very insular view of the body as a biological being (see Box 3.5). The beliefs, goals and knowledge required for the medical model have several limitations. It places an emphasis on cure not caring, which places nurses in a subservient position to doctors. This may in turn encourage nurses not to value the aspects of the patient that do not fit within the medical model and subsequently reduce care to lists of tasks to perform rather than holistic packages of care carefully worked out between nurse and patient.

You may tell a patient that they have asthma and that the 'cure' is a regime of inhaled drugs but other factors can interfere with the treatment. These may include:

- environmental factors such as pollution and allergens
- attitudes to chronic disease
- skills in administering treatment: dexterity, sight, memory
- values about health

Box 3.5 **The medical model**

Beliefs: man is a biological being whose integrity is disturbed by disease.

Goal: cure disease through medical treatment.

Knowledge: Biological sciences such as physiology, pathology and microbiology, and pharmacology.

- age
- ability to adapt to a new lifestyle
- extent of other disabilities
- level of education
- knowledge about the physiology of the body
- cultural beliefs about ill health
- ability to pay for expensive drugs and equipment
- ability to travel regularly for check ups

Developing a Framework for a Particular Area of Practice

There are several types of nursing models that have been developed but these are often more applicable to the institutional setting. Roper's original model was developed in response to changes in nursing between 1940 and 1970. It is centred around the activities of daily living, gives due consideration to a lifetime span from conception to death and incorporates a dependence to dependence continuum. It is a nursing model which suggests that the living person requires help with or takes part in four groups of activities, namely 'daily living', 'preventing', 'comforting' and 'seeking' activities (Roper, 1976). Despite the preventative and seeking aspects of this model, many practical interpretations of this model modify it to reflect nursing problems as opposed to patients problems. Most of them focus specifically on an illness to health continuum rather than take as their central tenet the restoration of equilibrium between the systems that are necessary in chronic disease management.

Dorothea Orem's (1991) model of nursing addressed the issue of patients' responsibility for their own health in her self care model. The beliefs that underpin this model are that individuals have self care needs and that they have the right to meet these needs if it is at all possible. Self care is a deliberate action that has as its purpose the meeting of individual requirements for effective living. Self care is learned behaviour; its development is aided by intellectual curiosity, by instruction and supervision from others, and by experience in performing self care measures. Its goals are to meet self care needs, either through supporting the patient in meeting his own self care needs, through enabling a relative or friend to be the self care agent, or through the nurse acting as the self care agent.

The knowledge centres on self care, that is, those actions which people take in order to function as a whole human being; Orem identified eight (see Box 3.6).

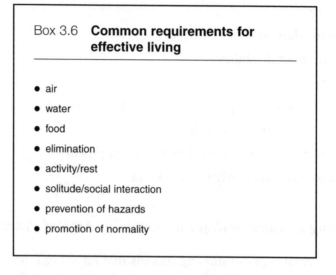

Box 3.6 **Common requirements for effective living**

- air
- water
- food
- elimination
- activity/rest
- solitude/social interaction
- prevention of hazards
- promotion of normality

These common requirements are affected by a wide variety of factors that are identified as the features that make an individual unique. The influencing factors are an integral part of the assessment so that an acceptable plan of care can be negotiated with the patient. The factors are all influences on self care ability and performance in relation to the requirements for effective living (see Box 3.7).

Life changes may be developmental, as in the progression from birth to death and the consequent effects of ageing. Or they may be changes that may cause problems at any time such as the loss of a job or relatives, poor educational opportunities, oppressive living conditions, poor health or disability and the subsequent change in status that this may bring. The following case study epitomises the features of this model.

'Maud' – a Case Study

Maud was born in 1930 in London and was an only child. Her relationship with her father was poor as he was in the RAF and frequently away. When Maud was 21 she married Ron, an electrician who she had known for five years. They had two children, born in 1954 and 1959 respectively. Just before their second child was born, the family moved to a rural area in East Anglia. As the children grew up Maud found employment as an optician's receptionist. In 1970, after years of heavy smoking and drinking, her husband collapsed and died of a heart attack. During this time, and in the

```
┌─────────────────────────────────────────────────────────┐
│                                                           │
│   Box 3.7   Influencing factors                           │
│   ──────────────────────────────────────────             │
│                                                           │
│   Skills              Knowledge of conditions             │
│                                                           │
│   Values              Promoting health and well-being     │
│                                                           │
│   Beliefs             Maturity                            │
│                                                           │
│   Habits              Motivation                          │
│                                                           │
│   Culture             Life cycle stages                   │
│                                                           │
│   Environment         Life change events                  │
│                                                           │
│   Knowledge of self   Health state                        │
│                                                           │
└─────────────────────────────────────────────────────────┘
```

next nine years, Maud was devastated, frightened and was very lonely until she met and married her second husband.

In November 1997, Maud began to feel 'not right'. She said she felt increasingly tired and listless, and started to feel sick in the day time and had an incredible thirst, especially at night. Her husband prompted her to go to the doctor where a diagnosis of non-insulin dependent diabetes was made. An appointment was made at the diabetic clinic where the following nursing assessment was made using Orem's model.

Air

Maud began smoking regularly 10 cigarettes a day when she moved to a small rural town in East Anglia at the age of 31. This was influenced by the stress of the move and looking for a job to supplement her husband's income. Her husband had smoked since the age of 19, smoking approximately 30–40 cigarettes a day by the time he was 25 years old. Her husband's death in 1970, sole care of her two sons, and subsequent remarriage (which resulted in her living with her mother-in-law) were such stressful times, that she never addressed her smoking. However, in 1995 Maud decided to give up smoking, encouraged by her second husband. Unfortunately this led to Maud putting on 20 kgs in weight, which made her feel tired and listless, especially in summer. As she lives at the bottom of a steep hill she found it increasingly difficult, due to breathlessness, to walk up it daily, so she restricted her shopping to once a week. Maud has a history of bronchitis but there is no family history of asthma or hay fever and Maud does not suffer from these conditions. Maud's blood pressure was 150/88 mmHg.

Water

Maud describes herself as a 'teetotaller' – alcohol irritates her stomach. Maud suffers from dyspepsia and requires regular antacids to relieve her heartburn. She drinks approximately eight cups a day of tea but does not enjoy coffee or plain water.

Food

Maud describes her diet as a little 'topsy turvy'. She does not always eat breakfast, but if she does it consists of cereal or white bread, butter and jam. Twice a week she would have a fried breakfast with her husband. Dinner would be anything from meat pies, rice dishes, fried fish, sausages, bacon and stews, all with plenty of fresh vegetables, as her husband has an allotment. Dessert would be homemade fruit pies or fruit and cream. Tea would always be white bread sandwiches with prawns, cheese, ham or bacon followed by cakes, biscuits or her favourite ice cream. Maud especially loved chocolate and strawberry creams. Maud's weight was 89 kg and height of 1.61 m gave her a body mass index of $33.56 \, kg/m^2$.

Elimination

Maud has suffered from irregular bouts of constipation since 1959. She has taken a mild laxative since 1965, which she requires regularly for her bowels to be open every two days. Maud's urinalysis was positive to sugar, which was reflected in her blood results of 18.4 mmol and a high HBA1c of 11.7 mmol.

Activity and Rest

Maud spends much of her time within her home. She is a house-proud woman, always ensuring that her house is clean and tidy despite her constant tiredness. She enjoys reading especially Catherine Cookson's novels and new recipes. Her ability to read was not affected by her visual acuity of 12/6 in her right eye and 60/6 in her left eye. She describes herself as a 'great sleeper' who likes to get up with her husband at 6.00 am and go to bed about 10 pm.

Solitude and Social Interaction

As Maud's husband spends his days at his allotment, she spends much of her time alone. She enjoys going to car boot sales with her friends on

Sundays to look for cheap novels and a good bargain. Neither she or her husband drive so they rarely go out in the evenings. However, they enjoy each other's company and make special dinners on Tuesdays and Saturdays as a treat to themselves. Maud has five grandchildren and another one on the way. She sees her grandchildren most weekends as she has maintained a close relationship with both of her sons.

Perception of Diagnosis

Maud's attitude to her diabetes, is remarkably positive and proactive. Following her diagnosis, she explained, that after her initial tears, she thought 'well it isn't the "other" (meaning cancer) and so I should feel lucky, so get on with it'. She admitted she knows little about diabetes and to feeling scared about her diagnosis at first as she had images of her elderly aunt who was on insulin therapy and had multiple complications of blindness and below knee amputation, but she did know that her control had been poor, ignoring a lot of advice she had been given. Maud's feet were in good condition with lower limb pulses, reflexes and sensation to stimuli present. Maud has a friend who has diabetes, which is diet controlled, and although they have never discussed her condition – Maud knows she always appears well and happy. Her husband and her sons were very supportive on learning of her diagnosis and read the handouts and discussed her diet plan with her.

From this assessment it is clear that Maud is an independent and self-caring person who is keen to develop her understanding of diabetes and to be fully involved in the management of her condition. Within each of the common requirements for effective living are features that will influence her ability to comply with a care plan. Her intellectual capacity and previous knowledge of the condition necessitate a clear and realistic teaching component. Maud will need support in her decision to stop smoking, especially as her previous smoking history was stress related. Another important feature of her plan is to lose weight and this may also trigger her smoking behaviour, as she felt quite certain that giving up smoking had precipitated her weight gain. Her supportive family and ability to anticipate the 'problems' of diabetes ensured that with the support of the healthcare team she would be able to live as normal a lifestyle as she had prior to her diagnosis.

To develop a model of practice requires a representation of all the disciplines within the team that interact with the patient. If a more equal partnership with the users of the service is to be arrived at then consumer representation should be elicited in this exercise. In this model all members of the team must be able to recognize the limitations and strengths of the individual within his or her own environment. This together with the patient's family history and motivation are key features of a self care model.

Conclusion

Making the process of nursing explicit to patients and to other members of the healthcare team is vital for the coordinated delivery of health care. Proactive assessment is a critical stage in encouraging patients to take back responsibility for their own health.

4

Asthma Assessment

ALISON PARKER

Asthma is a very common disease that is difficult to define. Box 4.1 demonstrates a simple definition from Barnes and Godfrey (1995). A more comprehensive description would include reference to the underlying pathology as well as the reversibility and variability of airflow obstruction, for example from the International Consensus Report on the Diagnosis and Management of Asthma (Bousquet and Michel, 1992) (see also Box 4.2).

Understanding the concept of asthma as a variable disease is important because the basis of good asthma management lies in the ability to interpret

---

Box 4.1 **Asthma – a simple definition**

Asthma is a syndrome characterised by airflow obstruction, which varies markedly, both spontaneously and with treatment.

Source: Barnes and Godfrey, 1995.

Box 4.2 **Asthma – underlying pathology**

Asthma is a chronic inflammatory disease of the airways in which many cells play a role, in particular mast cells and eosonophils. In susceptible individuals, this inflammation causes symptoms that are usually associated with widespread but variable airflow obstruction that is often reversible either spontaneously or with treatment and causes an associated increase in the airway responsiveness to a variety of stimuli.

Source: Bousquet and Michel, 1992.

the symptoms and degree of morbidity that the underlying inflammatory condition is causing and tailoring the treatment and education to the particular patient. Over recent years, the management of asthma has increasingly emphasized the use of anti-inflammatory drugs. This is because studies (Beasley *et al.*, 1989; Bousquet *et al.*, 1990; Laitinen *et al.*, 1985, 1993) conducted since the 1980s, have shown that even in mild, quiescent, asymptomatic asthma, inflammatory changes are apparent in the airways.

Pathological Changes in Asthma

The early features of the inflammatory processes in asthma are usually reversible. The process is due to a variety of factors including:

- epithelial disruption and shedding of the airway epithelium
- infiltration of the mucosa and submucosa by inflammatory cells, in particular eosonophils, neutrophils, T-lymphocytes, macrophages and mast cells
- the inflammatory cells release a variety of mediators, which in turn cause smooth muscle contraction, further plasma leakage, oedema and hyper-responsiveness of the airways
- increased secretions into the lumen of the airways. Typically these secretions contain excess sticky mucous and inflammatory cells, in particular mast cells and shed epithelium; these cells 'plug' the smaller airways
- in the subepithelium further damage occurs with vasodilation leading to plasma leakage and oedema, hyperplasia of the mucous glands and goblet cells, smooth muscle hypertrophy and basement membrane thickening
- cysteinyl leukotrienes are very potent bronchoconstrictors, with a much greater effect than histamine or platelet activating factors (Sampson and Holgate, 1998). They are synthesised by mast cells, which recruit eosonophils into the area. They also increase mucous secretion in the airways, which slows the cilia thus leading to decreased mucous clearance.

Combinations of all the above symptoms lead to airway narrowing (see Figure 4.1).

Asthma is precipitated by a number of different factors. It is now known that some people have a genetic predisposition to developing the disease (Postma *et al.*, 1995) and that under certain conditions, for example allergy,

Figure 4.1   Asthma – multiple inflammatory mediators

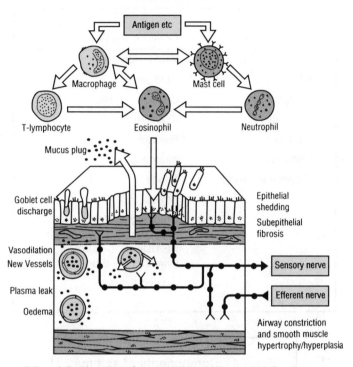

Source: Barnes, P. J. and Godfrey, S. *Asthma*, 1995, Martin Dunitz Ltd, London

viruses or certain occupational exposure, asthma can be provoked. Individual factors are known as inducers. Inducers cause airway inflammation, which alone may cause symptoms but also leads to an increase in the reactivity of the airways which is known as airway hyper-responsiveness, sometimes described as 'twitchy airways'. As can be seen from Box 4.3 there can be some cross over between inducers and triggers. Nerve endings exposed by epithelial damage become hyper-responsive to a variety of triggers, leading to airway narrowing and the infiltration of inflammatory cells which in turn release mediators thus causing further inflammation. Again, in turn, this causes smooth muscle contraction, increased mucus secretion and oedema, and further stimulation of sensory nerve endings. Hence, the inflammatory cycle is perpetuated (see Box 4.4).

Bronchoconstriction is usually reversible either in time or with drugs. However, evidence shows that under-treated asthma might lead to

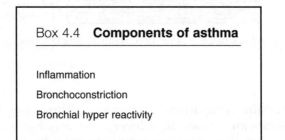

Box 4.3 **Asthma-inducers and triggers**

Possible inducers	Common triggers
Genetic factors	Viral infections
Atopy	Cold air
Allergies	Cigarette smoke
Occupational	Exercise
Exposure	Pollution
Infections	Allergens
Maternal smoking	Foods
	Stress
	Drugs eg. β-blockers including eye drops, aspirin, NSAIDs Non-steroidal anti inflammatory drugs
	Inhaled therapy

Box 4.4 **Components of asthma**

Inflammation

Bronchoconstriction

Bronchial hyper reactivity

irreversible airway damage which manifests as basement membrane thickening, smooth muscle hyperplasia and an increase in the total wall thickness, the so called 'airway wall remodelling' as described by Redington and Howarth (1997).

Symptoms

Changes in the airways of an asthmatic lead to the presence of symptoms in varying degrees, though not always directly reflective of the amount of

---

Box 4.5 **Symptoms of asthma**

Cough	Often the predominant and sometimes only symptom in children
Wheeze	Should be on expiration, caused by forcing air out through narrowed airways
Dyspnoea	Very common, shortness of breath
Chest tightness	Can be confused with cardiac problems in the elderly

---

inflammation present. The following table of symptoms may occur singly or in any combination (see Box 4.5).

Signs

Signs of asthma are often not present, but may include:

- chest wall deformity in people who have chronically under-treated or severe asthma. Harrison's Sulci is a physical sign of airway obstruction where there is a dip either side of the breastbone in the lower ribs. Associated changes of the breastbone, pectus carinatum or excavatum, may also be observed. These deformities tend to be seen in young children with malleable chest walls or in older patients who may have had asthma in childhood prior to the advent of inhaled steroids.
- hyperinflated chest with the use of accessory muscles present in acute asthma
- audible wheeze on expiration

Many people with symptoms of asthma may appear to be well during the day with a chest that sounds clear, which is why an important factor in diagnosis and management is the history taking, both as a part of the initial and the subsequent assessments.

Assessment

The initial clinic assessment is extremely important, providing the first vital clues to a complete picture of the patient: needs, expectations, current

---

Box 4.6 **Aims of asthma management**

- To abolish symptoms
- To restore normal or best possible airway function
- To reduce the risk of severe attacks
- To enable normal growth in children
- To minimise absence from school or work
- In achieving these goals, to avoid the side effects of therapy

---

morbidity, preconceived ideas and level of knowledge about the disease. It should give sufficient information to enable the assessor to judge where and what level of investigations or treatment should be initiated. Campbell *et al.* (1995) maintain that a broader paradigm than the traditional medical model should be considered when assessing patients with asthma. Therefore, the use of Orem's self care nursing model as a framework for assessment, education and promotion of guided self management would fit well with the principles of asthma management (see Box 4.6).

The principle philosophy being that most people wish to be self caring and that by a process of learning and development, facilitated by the team, the person will, within certain parameters and within their ability, be able to function normally in spite of having a chronic disease. It is useful to consider what information is required under Orem's nine categories of self care. Even though they may not all be pertinent to each disease process, it is a structured approach which examines areas perhaps not traditionally recognized as being relevant (see Table 4.1).

Taking a Formal History

Part of the initial assessment will include a formal history. How much one may obtain on a first visit is variable and depends on whether it is an emergency, a new diagnosis, the age of the patient and the attitude portrayed. Information that should be included is summarised in Box 4.7.

Examination

Included in a first visit will be a physical assessment. There are various ways to obtain information which can be classified under the following

Table 4.1 Orem's self care model for asthmatics

Orem's category		Comment
Air	Expected peak expiratory flow rate (PEFR) Actual PEFR Best ever PEFR if known	
Environment	Rural/industrial Occupation Housing Smoker either active or passive Pollens Pets Known atopic Symptoms	In adults occupation is very important especially any recent job change Particularly in children's symptoms Where are the pets kept? Previous rhinitis or eczema? Cough, wheeze, shortness of breath, chest tightness
Water	Adequate	Especially during an acute exacerbation if mouth breathing or in COPD
Food	Known trigger factors: red wine dairy products fizzy drinks	Eating small nutritional meals for those with acute or severe chronic asthma with an irreversible element
Elimination	Potential problem of retention or constipation in high dose usage of anti cholinergics Sputum production	Stress incontinence can be a problem in coughers which only can be determined by asking Usually little but large quantity may be more indicative of other respiratory disease
Activity/rest	Night-time symptoms are classic in uncontrolled asthma Normal daily activities such as housework or stair climbing may be affected as exercise means different things to different people. Sexuality	Does the patient or carer appear tired? Lack of sleep affects growth in children, the ability to concentrate in the day, so affecting schoolwork Adults may be underachieving at work or having time off to care for a child

Table 4.1 Continued

Orem's category		Comment
	may be affected due to symptoms, again, information that may not be readily proffered	Symptoms while exercising, but shortness of breath, especially in the elderly, may indicate heart failure especially if they have swollen ankles
Solitude and social interaction	Work, hobbies, stress and social life	
	Days off work or school due to exacerbations	May be curtailed by embarrassment due to symptoms, or inability to cope with smoky atmospheres in public places
	Personal details	What support do they have from family, friends or peer group?
	Family history of atopy	May be due to overprotection from parents or carer
	Lack of personal space	Acceptance of symptoms as normal especially in the elderly who may view them as part of the normal ageing process
	Social isolation	Recognized as an important contributing factor in asthma deaths (Mohan et al., 1996)
Prevention of hazards	Smoking	Avoidance of active or passive smoking
	Life threatening asthma → avoidance of trigger factors where possible	Appropriate recognition and appropriate treatment of
	Detecting drugs either as precipitators or aggravators of pre-existing asthma	Carry reliever always
		Investigating/exploring beliefs or worries re. drugs/side effects
		Acceptance of disease
Promotion of normality	May depend on age at diagnosis	Enabling normal growth in children
	Use of preventer to enable normal lifestyle	Freedom from side effects of treatment while controlling symptoms
	Avoidance of illness	

Box 4.7 **Formal history framework**

Personal Details

Smoking History → Active/Passive

Asthma: past history

Medical History

---

three headings:

Observation:

- colour
- cough
- expiratory wheeze
- shortness of breath
- anxiety
- use of accessory muscles
- nicotine finger staining or smell of smoke
- respiratory rate
- happy/well

Measurement:

- PEFR
- lung function – spirometry
- symptom chart
- height and weight
- blood pressure
- urinalysis
- use of reliever medication
- repeat prescriptions
- subjective that is, well being as reported

Interviewing:

- questioning skills
- using open and closed questions
- discussion with carer or relative

Diagnosis

Diagnosis of asthma is made on both objective and subjective measurements along with response to treatment. In adults and children above the age of five the diagnosis is usually easier because, generally, the majority will be able to use a peak flow meter or spirometer if available, which aids the detection of the variability of airway tone that underpins the diagnosis. It also differentiates from other lung conditions, where fixed airway obstruction may be present, as in chronic obstructive pulmonary disease (COPD). More complicated lung function can be measured in hospital if there is doubt about the diagnosis, for example histamine or methacholine challenge testing and controlled exercise testing. However, 95 per cent of asthma is diagnosed and managed in general practice with only the more severe or difficult to manage cases being referred to secondary care.

In very young children, particularly the under 2s, diagnosis can be more difficult. Suspicion should be raised when children repeatedly present with 'chest infections' or nocturnal cough. There is some concern that the presence of a cough alone, in the absence of measurable airway obstruction, does not indicate asthma (Chang *et al.*, 1998). A careful history should be taken of the frequency of symptoms and details of any first-degree family history of atopic disease. It is very useful to use a scoring system to record symptoms of wheeze and cough over a period of time along with frequency of use and the response to any bronchodilator therapy prescribed. An example of a scoring system is given in Box 4.8 (adapted from original work by Dr Ian Charlton, Southampton). Reasons for employing this strategy are:

- it is difficult for a parent to remember how many nights they were wakened by a child with nocturnal cough or wheeze during the past week, never mind the previous month
- it provides some subjective measurement to frequency and morbidity of the disease
- it focuses the parent to determine to what degree the symptoms are present. It is very easy to become complacent in the presence of a persistent background cough, perhaps insufficient to waken a child, but may cause damage from low-grade chronic symptoms.

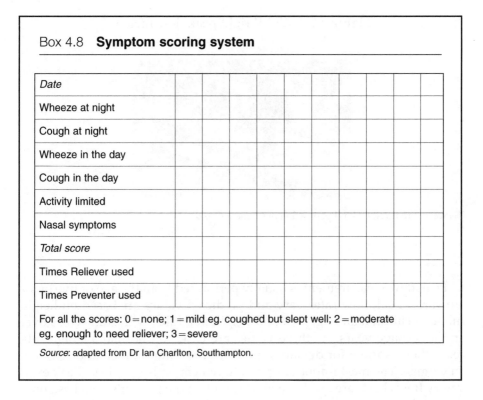

Box 4.8 **Symptom scoring system**

Date										
Wheeze at night										
Cough at night										
Wheeze in the day										
Cough in the day										
Activity limited										
Nasal symptoms										
Total score										
Times Reliever used										
Times Preventer used										

For all the scores: 0 = none; 1 = mild eg. coughed but slept well; 2 = moderate eg. enough to need reliever; 3 = severe

Source: adapted from Dr Ian Charlton, Southampton.

- it assists in the assessment of response to treatment
- it aids planning guided self (or parent) management
- in children it is important to distinguish between chronic persistent symptoms and episodic symptoms caused by viral triggers, as the management is quite different (Silverman, 1997)

Tools of Assessment

The most commonly used tool in asthma assessment is the peak flow meter, which provides an objective measurement of lung function. It measures the maximum flow of air expelled from the lungs in litres per minute maintained for 10 ms from a forced manoeuvre. The result is effort dependent and, therefore, can only be used in co-operative patients. There are a variety of peak flow meters available. The preference is that for reproducibility and consistency the patient's own meter is used but if this is not possible at least the same type of meter, for example Wrights mini peak flow (see Figure 4.2).

Figure 4.2   Mini-Wright peak flow meters

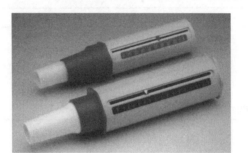

Source: Reproduced by kind permission of Clement Clarke

Peak flow measurement is usually performed from the age of five or six upwards. Peak flow rates vary and predicted values are based on height alone in children and age, sex and height in adults, with some cross over in the teenage years. As these values are based on normal average subjects, there is room for deviation of up to 1001/min in men and 851/min in women. The most important point to remember is that these Peak expiratory flow charts are used as a guide and that the patient's own best, once it is achieved, is used as a basis for on-going monitoring and assessment of control (see Figure 4.3).

The best way to teach use of the peak flow meter is to demonstrate the technique to the patient (see Box 4.9). Peak flow meters are portable and available on prescription. They are used initially in the diagnosis and subsequently in the management of asthma. Single readings are of little value because of the diurnal variation of the disease. Therefore, it is important to have serial recordings to enable the assessor to detect the 15 per cent or more variability, which is indicative of asthma. Certain circumstances, other than time of day, may influence the readings, such as time of year, influence of trigger factors, presence of other lung disease such as chronic obstructive airways disease, or incorrect technique. It is essential to determine the last time a bronchodilator was used.

Other Peak Flow-Based Diagnostic Tests

Normal diurnal variation in non-asthmatic people is 5 to 8 per cent. An increase of 15 per cent or more from baseline is generally accepted as diagnostic of asthma.

Figure 4.3 Peak expiratory flow in normal adults

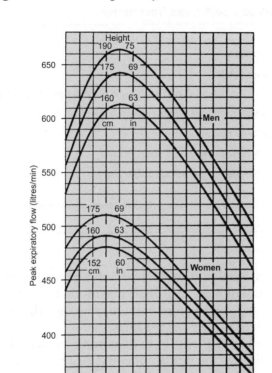

Source: This figure was first published in the *British Medical Journal*. I. Gregg and A. J. Nunn. 'The Normal Peak Flow in Adults', 1989; **298**: 1068–70 and is reproduced by permission of the *British Medical Journal*.

Reversibility Test:

1. Measure and record the patient's PEFR

2. Give salbutamol 200 mcgs or terbutaline 500 mcgs via a large volume spacer

3. Remeasure and record the PEFR after 15 minutes

4. Work out the percentage increase by the following Formula

$$\frac{\text{Highest PEFR} - \text{Lowest PEFR}}{\text{Highest PEFR}} \times 100$$

5. An increase of 15 to 20 per cent is diagnostic of asthma

Box 4.9 **How to use a peak flow meter**

---

1. Stand up if possible.

2. Place the cursor on zero.

3. Take a deep breath, place teeth and lips around the mouthpiece, to make a tight seal.

4. Blow hard and fast, noting the number at which the cursor rests.

5. Return the cursor to zero.

6. Repeat twice and obtain three readings.

7. Plot the highest of the three readings on the chart.

Source: Reproduced with permission from the National Asthma and Respiratory Training Centre.

As asthma is a reversible disease a negative reversibility test does not exclude it. The patient may be at their maximum bronchodilation, or the extent of the oedema and inflammation may be such that bronchodilators alone are insufficient to alter the readings.

In the presence of symptoms or to determine whether this is reversible or fixed airway disease, the next step would be a steroid reversibility test. This requires the patient to have a daily dose of prednisolone 30 to 40 mgs for an adult for between two and three weeks while maintaining serial peak flow recordings at home on a diary card. All patients requiring a steroid course should first have their blood pressure recorded, urinalysis done and any relevant history of gastric ulcers determined, due to the possibility of side effects. If available, the use of spirometry pre- and post-steroid course is useful, as the smaller increase in values measurable in FEV1 and FVC in possible COPD with reversibility is more useful.

Exercise Test

It is estimated that 80 per cent of asthmatics have some degree of exercise induced asthma (EIA) (Cochrane *et al.*, 1996), and although the majority will have symptoms at other times, there are some people whose asthma is truly only exercise induced. These people will only have the diagnosis proven by showing a fall from their baseline PEFR reading of 15 per cent or more. The test is best done outside, as the cooler air conditions along with the hyperventilation of exercise and the drying out of the airway mucosa are what are thought to be the mechanism of the condition.

Exercise as a trigger produces immediate symptoms but does not give rise to a delayed onset or late response because it does not increase the inflammatory process. However, in a similar way conditions of cold dry air can trigger symptoms of increased bronchial hyper reactivity in asthmatics whose asthma is not well controlled.

Exercise Test:

1. Measure and record the PEFR.
2. Run for six minutes (preferably outside) and record the PEFR.
3. Repeat the recording of the PEFR three times at five minute intervals.
4. A 15 per cent or more fall in PEFR from baseline indicates exercise-induced asthma.

Any doubt in the diagnosis in children or adults requires referral to a respiratory physician or paediatrician. In children unable to use a peak flow meter then a symptom scoring chart should be used as discussed previously.

Recording of Information

It will depend on your practice and personal choice how information is recorded. A variety of assessment cards are available from drug companies, or the National Asthma and Respiratory Training Centre have their own Gold Card. Some people prefer to design their own or to use the Tayside Assessment Stamp (see Figure 4.4) directly in the notes and can be used for ongoing monitoring and audit.

Asthma Drugs

The majority of asthma medication has been developed as inhaled therapy and it is the preferred route of treatment (see Table 4.2). Inhaled medication tends to work more quickly, minimises the dosage and reduces the potential for side effects (Devices for inhalation will be discussed separately). There are two main groups of drugs used in the management of asthma, namely relievers and preventers (see Box 4.10).

Relievers

Relievers are drugs that give symptomatic relief by relaxing bronchial smooth muscle. They are short acting, and have no effect on the underlying inflammation.

Figure 4.4   Tayside assessment stamp

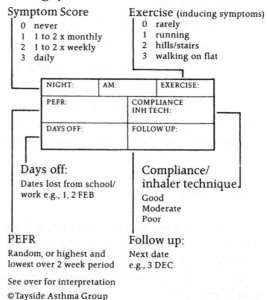

USING PATIENT RECORD STAMP

Fill in the blanks using this suggested scoring system.

Symptom Score
  0 never
  1 1 to 2 x monthly
  2 1 to 2 x weekly
  3 daily

Exercise (inducing symptoms)
  0 rarely
  1 running
  2 hills/stairs
  3 walking on flat

NIGHT:	AM:	EXERCISE:
PEFR:	COMPLIANCE INH TECH:	
DAYS OFF:	FOLLOW UP:	

Days off:
Dates lost from school/ work e.g., 1, 2 FEB

Compliance/ inhaler technique.
Good
Moderate
Poor

PEFR
Random, or highest and lowest over 2 week period

Follow up:
Next date e.g., 3 DEC

See over for interpretation
©Tayside Asthma Group

β_2 agonists:

Inhaled short acting β_2 agonists work by binding with the adrenergic receptors in the lung stimulating the β_2 receptors found mainly in the bronchial smooth muscle thus causing bronchodilation. They begin to work within two to three minutes and their effect lasts from four to six hours. They should be used on an as-required basis for the relief of symptoms, or before exercise to prevent the onset of exercise induced symptoms. There is evidence to suggest that if used in high dosage on a regular basis there is a degree of loss of bronchodilatory response and a rebound hyper-responsiveness of the airways if the drug is withheld (Cochrane *et al.*, 1996). The response to bronchodilators seems to be preserved if used in conjunction with inhaled steroid therapy.

Table 4.2 Asthma medication – summary of action and usage

Class	Generic name	Mode of action	Possible side effects	Delivery	Comment
Corticosteroids	*Inhaled* beclomathasone budesonide fluticasone	*Anti-inflammatory* Suppresses inflammatory cells and prevents their migration Reduces airway oedema Reduces mucous secretion Increases responsiveness of β receptors in smooth muscle	*Inhaled* Local- dysphonia (hoarseness) and oral candida (thrush) High doses >1000 mcgs daily may, over time, cause skin thinning and bruising and adrenal suppression	*Inhaled* A variety of inhalers see section on device selection	Local side effects can be minimized by the use of spacer devices and good oral hygiene Rinsing the mouth after inhaling steroids, washing the face of babies if using a face mask and having a drink of water after are all good preventive measures along with minimizing the dose to attain control.
	Oral prednisolone prednesol		*Oral* Long term use – high likelihood of: osteoporosis cataracts diabetes obesity hypertension adrenal suppression muscle weakness skin thinning and bruising	*Oral* Tablets enteric coated tablets soluble tablets	
Cromones		*Anti-inflammatory* Inhibits action and release of mediators from inflammatory cells particularly mast cells	Cough on inhalation	Inhaled only	Bitter taste from sodium cromoglycate Possible problem with compliance as tds or qds dosage nedocromil has mint taste takes 4–6 weeks to take effect

Table 4.2 Continued

Class	Generic name	Mode of action	Possible side effects	Delivery	Comment
Leukotriene inhibitor antagonists	montelukast zafirlukast	*Anti-inflammatory* Inhibits the release of leukotrienes Reduces mucous production Reduces vascular leakage and oedema Increases cilial activity and mucous clearance Reduces inflammatory cells	Rare Headache	Oral only Tablets	
Methylxanthines	theophyllines	Bronchodilation Possible anti-inflammatory effect	Multiple nausea vomiting cardiac arrythmia enuresis	*Oral* Available as slow release tablets Syrup Intravenous use in severe asthma	Possibility of over-dosage in intravenous usage if already on oral drug
β₂ agonists Short acting	salbutamol terbutaline	Bronchodilation by stabilizing the mast cells stimulating the β₂ receptors thus relaxing bronchial smooth muscle	*Common* Headache tremor tachycardia anxiety/restlessness *Less Common* Hypokalaemia Hypoxaemia rare side effect, usually from nebulising and causing a mismatch	*Oral* Syrup requires high doses Slow release tablets *Inhaled* Metered dose inhaler and dry powder Also nebuliser solutions though side effects increase on higher doses	Subsequent increase in side effects Rapid onset of action 2–3 minutes Duration of action of 4–6 hours Can have a tachyphylactic effect therefore should be a

			of O_2 and CO_2 due to pulmonary vasodilation	*Parenteral* Subcutaneous bricanyl	prn drug except in an acute exacerbation Over reliance is dangerous and implicated in the increase in asthma deaths of the 1980s Given in acute severe asthma where other methods have failed
β₂ agonists Long-acting	salmeterol formoterol	Inhaled bronchodilatory effect and protection from bronchoconstriction for 12 hours	As for short-acting bronchodilators	*Inhaled* Salmeterol Formoterol	Salmeterol slower onset of action of up to 20 minutes Formoterol onset 2–3 minutes Not for use in an acute attack Useful for protection against exercise induced symptoms and in nocturnal asthma Must be used in conjunction with an anti-inflammatory Has steroid-sparing property
	bambec	Oral long acting reliever for 24 hour effect			
Anticholinergics	ipratropium bromide oxitropium bromide	Work by blocking the muscarinic receptors thereby reducing vagal tone and preventing bronchoconstriction	May cause dry mouth In rare cases causes urinary retention Occasionally causes paradoxical bronchoconstriction Can cause glaucoma from nebulising	*Only available as inhaled drug coma* Available as metered dose inhaler, and nebuliser solution. Ipratropium as a dry powder	*Special precaution* If nebulising a mouthpiece be used to protect the eyes and prevent the development of glaucoma Useful drug in the young Often most effective bronchodilator for use in COPD

Table 4.2 Continued

Class	Generic name	Mode of action	Possible side effects	Delivery	Comment
Combined therapy	combivent	Combined effect of both classes of drugs	As above	*Inhaled only* Metered dose inhaler and as a solution for nebuliser	Useful for COPD and more severe asthma
	seretide	Combined fluticasone and salmeterol		Available in dry powder and CFC free metered dose inhaler	Useful for assisting compliance in asthma

---

Box 4.10 **Asthma drugs**

Relievers	*Preventers*
β_2 Agonists	Mast cell stabilisers
Anticholinergics	Inhaled steroids
Theophyllines	Leukotriene antagonists
	Oral steroids

Common side effects of β_2 agonists are tremor, tachycardia, headache and feelings of anxiety. In people unable to tolerate the side effects of one β_2 agonist, changing to a different preparation often helps. Long acting β_2 agonists, for example salmeterol maintain a bronchodilator effect for between 12 and 18 hours and are used twice a day as an add-on therapy to a steroid inhaler. Their use is indicated for patients who are using high dose inhaled steroids or having breakthrough nocturnal or exercise induced symptoms despite being on an adequate dose of a preventer therapy. The onset of action is slower than that of short acting β_2 agonists; they are, therefore, not suitable for use in acute management.

Anticholinergics

In the lungs there is a constant action from the parasympathetic pathway, which gives the lungs tone and helps keep the airways from collapsing. Anticholinergics work by binding with the muscarinic receptors, thus blocking the parasympathetic transmitter effect of acetylcholine at the bronchoconstrictor nerve endings, thereby preventing bronchoconstriction.

The mode of action is slower than that of β_2 agonists, having some effect from around 15 minutes and taking around 40 minutes to attain maximum bronchodilation. Ipratroprium bromide (atrovent) is a short acting anticholinergic with duration of between 6 and 8 hours. Oxytropium bromide (oxivent) is long acting with an action of around 12 hours. Anticholinergics are particularly useful in the management of severe asthma or COPD where reversibility is often better with anticholinergics acting on vagal tone. They are sometimes used in very young children with asthma in whom the response to β_2 agonists may be suboptimal.

Combined therapy

Combined therapy of salbutamol and atrovent is sometimes used. It may prove more effective for the relief of symptoms in COPD where the combination of the two drugs may have a synergistic effect in a different disease profile where the treatment aim is to maximise bronchodilation.

Seretide

A more recent addition to combined therapy at level three of the guidelines is an inhaled steroid and long acting β_2 agonist. This may make an impression on compliance by giving better control in a single inhaler with less cost and time to the patient.

Methylxanthines

Methylxanthines are a group of drugs that are not available via the inhaled route. They are either given orally or intravenously in severe asthma. They are drugs that, if used in the high doses required to facilitate bronchodilation, that is 12–20 mg/litre plasma concentration, have a high side effect profile. Recently there has been evidence showing that they may have some anti-inflammatory effect in lower dosages with plasma concentrations of 5–10 mg/litre (Markham and Faulds, 1998; Aizawa *et al.*, 2000). Over the last few years with the wider use of inhaled steroids and long acting bronchodilators they have been used less frequently.

Although these drugs have been around a long time, their mode of action is not fully understood. However, they may reduce inflammatory mediators and some intracellular changes effect bronchodilation. Side effects include nausea and vomiting, enuresis in children, restlessness, cardiac arrhythmia and gastric irritation. The plasma level of the drug can be altered by a variety of factors and this can lead to complications and toxicity. See Table 4.3.

Preventers

The term preventer is used to describe the action of drugs that reduce the chronic inflammation which underpins the disease process in asthma. Until this year, there were only two classes of drugs that fitted this description, cromones (non-steroidal anti-inflammatory drugs), or inhaled

Table 4.3 Methylxanthines and drug interactions

Drug	Increased plasma level	Decreased plasma level
allopurinol	✓	
carbemazepine		✓
cimetidine	✓	
erythromycin	✓	
oral contraceptives	✓	
phenobarbitone		✓
phenytoin		✓
propranolol	✓	
Other factors		
children		✓
elderly	✓	
cardiac failure	✓	
liver disease	✓	

steroids. Recently a new class of anti-inflammatory drug has been introduced, known as cysteinyl leukotriene antagonists.

Cromones

Otherwise known as mast cell stabilisers, these work by blocking the release of inflammatory mediators that predispose and enhance the inflammation in the airways of asthmatics. Cromones are placed in treatment guidelines (BTS, 1997) for mild to moderate asthma. In children they have to be used three to four times daily and usually twice daily for adults. They can take between four to six weeks to be effective, and are only effective in a small number of asthmatics (Rees and Price, 1995). Inhaled steroids are now the first line therapy for most asthmatics due to their high safety profile and greater efficacy (Levy *et al.*, 1997). Sodium cromoglycate (intal) is available as an inhaled drug for children and as nedocromil sodium (tilade) for adults.

Inhaled Steroids

Inhaled steroids are the mainstays of asthma drug management. They work by suppressing inflammation, reducing vasodilation – which decreases plasma leakage and oedema – and inhibiting mucous secretion.

The drug binds with a glucocorticoid receptor. It then works within the cell to inhibit the production of a variety of cytokines and this in turn reduces the eosonophilic infiltration of the airways, which then further limits the production of other inflammatory mediators such as leukotrienes and prostaglandins. The reduction in inflammation, mucous secretion and oedema leads to a much less sensitive airway which then may revert to normal, in that cilia regrow on an intact epithelium thus reducing the exposure of the sensory nerve endings in the airway. The sensitivity of β_2 receptors also becomes enhanced.

Currently there are three inhaled corticosteroids available in this country: budesonide, beclomethasone dipropionate and fluticasone proprionate. Although their make-up is slightly different in effect they have the same outcome. Fluticasone is twice as potent as beclomathasone and budesonide but is said to be less bio available. This means that the majority of the drug is excreted by the liver directly from the stomach without entering the systemic circulation and, therefore, has less potential for side effects. However with all inhaled drugs a percentage is absorbed directly from the lungs into the systemic circulation. Often it is possible to use fluticasone at half the dose of the other inhaled steroids to achieve the same effect.

Inhaled steroids do not have an immediate effect, they will begin to work within a few days of starting a twice daily dose, but may take up to four weeks to achieve maximum response, and several months to lose the hyper-reactivity, or 'twitchiness', of the airways in previously uncontrolled asthma.

Leukotriene Receptor Agonists

Leukotriene receptor agonists are a new class of drug to the UK and are yet to have their place set in national guidelines. They work on the inflammatory cascade and inhibit the release of cysteinyl leukotrienes by blocking their receptor sites, thereby reducing the inflammatory pool. In turn mucous production decreases; there is less vascular leakage, fewer inflammatory cells and greater cilial activity leading to less inflammation. There is evidence to suggest that airway hyper-responsiveness may be reduced (Sampson, 1996).

Currently there are two leukotriene receptor agonists. The first, montelukast (singulair) that is available for children from the age of two as a once daily 5 mg tablet, 10 mg for adults taken at night. Zafirlukast (accolate) is prescribable from the age of 12 as a twice a day tablet. While montelukast is recommended for use in mild to moderate asthma in addition to inhaled steroid therapy or as a mono therapy for exercise induced asthma, Zafirlukast is available as a first line therapy in mild to moderate asthma.

Inhaler Devices

One of the most fundamental aspects of good asthma management is the appropriate selection and use of inhaler devices. A simple study by Pool (1995) looked at inhaler technique and device appropriateness of 50 children newly referred, consecutively, to a paediatric asthma specialist nurse in Addenbrookes Hospital, Cambridge for help in managing difficult to control asthma. The outcome was that 48 of the 50 had an inhaler technique evaluated as being poor enough to detrimentally affect their asthma control. This may not have been the only factor involved. However, it highlights the scenario of increasing doses of medication and the potential increased risk of side effects, along with the expense of referral to secondary care and the increased risk of hospital admission for acute asthma, when a failure of a basic management skill in asthma care should have been addressed.

Device Selection

For the majority of people requiring medication for respiratory disease the inhaled route is preferred and recommended in the BTS (Guidelines on Asthma Management, 1997) for a variety of reasons:

- it is quick and efficient (if used correctly)
- uses small doses
- reduces the risk of side effects

When considering the devices most suitable for an individual, there are some basic criteria the health professional must apply and these are summarised in Box 4.11. Each of these areas is important, although cost from a health professional's point of view, will probably differ from that of a purchaser or pharmacist. (For guides to using inhalers see 'A guide to Asthma Inhalers' (Pearce, 1998).)

How do you measure cost in terms of emotional stress and increasing morbidity or loss of earnings experienced by the patient who may not have the correct drug or inhaler because they are deemed too expensive? It may, therefore, be useful to consider the cost implications of poor or inappropriate device selection in terms of hospital admissions and referral to

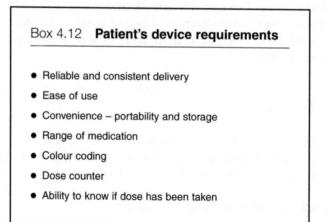

Box 4.11   **Basic considerations in device selection**

- Patient/carers ability
- Patients dexterity
- Patients age
- Inspiratory flow rate
- Tidal volume
- Ability to hold breath
- Acceptable to patient
- Cost

Box 4.12   **Patient's device requirements**

- Reliable and consistent delivery
- Ease of use
- Convenience – portability and storage
- Range of medication
- Colour coding
- Dose counter
- Ability to know if dose has been taken

secondary care because of poor control. Remembering that the most expensive inhaler device is the one that the patient does not use, Crompton (1998) reminds us that the user's specification of an inhaler may not match ours. Patients' perceptions regarding the need for treatment, their attitudes and preconceived ideas have to be addressed first and what qualities they feel are important need to be considered and discussed with the patient. The BTS (1997) guidelines recommend that patient preference is of primary importance when choosing a device. A summary of patient's device requirements is shown in Box 4.12.

The ideal inhalation device described by O'Connor (1996) would

> achieve maximum drug delivery to the lung without any oropharyngeal deposition or any potential for systemic absorption via non-pulmonary pathways. In addition

the device should be easy to use and teach, be acceptable to patients and prescribers alike, and have minimal local side effects resulting in overall enhanced compliance.

Asthma management has come a long way since the metered dose inhaler was introduced, but the ideal device does not yet exist. The summary given in Table 4.4 highlights the pros and cons of the different types along with any special recommendations for use.

Inhaler History

First introduced in the mid 1950s, the pressurised metered dose inhaler (pMDI) remains, in spite of more recent technical advances, the most commonly prescribed inhaler, probably due to its relative cheapness. It is estimated that at least 50 per cent of all patients with metered dose inhalers use them incorrectly (Hilton, 1990). Patients find them difficult to use and so do the educators (see Box 4.13 for guidelines on educational procedure). A simple exercise conducted prior to a Cambridge Asthma Group nurses meeting tested the inhaler technique of all those attending with the aid of an aerosol inhalation meter (AIMs). The result was that 40 per cent were unable to pass all three measured criteria, namely firing the device, correct inspiration and breath holding. This is not peculiar to asthma nurses in Cambridge and is upheld by work done by Seaton *et al.* (1992). This of course has a huge bearing on their ability to teach the technique to others.

In any inhaler what is important is the therapeutic dose or respirable fraction that actually reaches the lungs. This is measurable in microns. Work done by Stalhofen *et al.* (1980) has shown that between 2 and 5 microns (μm) are optimal, small enough to get to the airways and stay there. Under 2 μm they are exhaled and above 5 μm usually become lodged in the oropharynx with the potential, if it is an inhaled steroid, to cause side effects, either locally as oral thrush or dysphonia, or systemically if the patient is on a high dose and the excess is swallowed and absorbed. Various studies have shown that around 80 per cent of the total inhaled dose from an pMDI lodges in the oropharynx with round 10 per cent reaching the airways and 10 per cent being retained in the inhaler (Newman *et al.*, 1981, Pederson, 1987). The same studies show that the rate of inhalation affects the percentage deposition in the airways; a long slow inspiration followed by holding the breath for 10 seconds results in the highest deposition.

Another problem associated with the use of aerosol inhalers both in pMDI and breath actuated devices is the 'cold freon effect', where the effect of the 70-mph aerosol leaving the inhaler hits the oropharynx and causes the patient to stop inhaling, thereby preventing the dose reaching the lungs.

Table 4.4 Inhaler devices

Device	Inspiratory flow needed	Maximum deposition	Advantages	Disadvantages	Comment
Metered dose inhaler	20–40 liters/minute	15%	Cheap Portable Full range of therapies	Difficult to co-ordinate Poor deposition Cold freon effect No indication when empty No dose indicator	Unsuitable for under 12 years of age CFC free inhalers may need some dose adjustment Spacehaler has reduced the aerosol speed and reduces problems with impact and increases deposition
Breath actuated Autohaler	20–30 liters/minute		No need to co-ordinate actuation and inspiration Better deposition than MDI	Some cold freon effect Occasional problems with firing Click sometimes stops patients from completing the inhalation	
Easibreathe	25–30 litres/minute		Still reasonable cheap Easy to use and teach Portable/compact	No indication when empty No dose indicator	Useful from age six onwards
Large Volume Spacer	Variable	Variations in deposition can be up to 50% between spacer devices*	Allows delivery of inhaled drugs to all patients Reduces side effects from oropharyngeal	Cumbersome Not easily portable Compliance is not always good	For all ages including the very young if used with a face mask Ensure a portable bronchodilator is prescribed

Device	Inspiratory flow	Lung deposition	Advantages	Disadvantages	Comments
			deposition and absorption* Reduces side effects from tachycardia and bronchoconstriction Overcomes the problem of hand to lung co-ordination	Not all inhalers are compatible with the different spacers	for the over fives even if they need a spacer for their preventer Spacer should be washed and allowed to dry in the air to reduce static *Single* actuations only to be used Reduces or prevents the cold freon effect
Small volume spacer Aerochamber	Tidal breathing	Variable	More acceptable to babies Soft valves need only small respiratory effort Smaller volume advantageous up to 150 ml lung volume More portable than large spacers	May need larger drug dosage for therapeutic effect Expensive as not on prescription	See how to use spacers with babies and toddlers Drug needs to be inhaled in 10 seconds ** so one actuation followed by five tidal breaths is sufficient
Medium volume spacer Babyhaler					
Dry powder devices Spinhaler	30–60 litres/minute	6–12%	Portable	May have agglomeration of particles at high humidity May cause bronchoconstriction from powder	Single dose devices need an extra element of dexterity Only available for one drug
Rotahaler	30–60 litres/minute	6–11%	Portable No co-ordination required	Requires fast inspiration and may be more difficult to	

Table 4.4 Continued

Device	Inspiratory flow needed	Maximum deposition	Advantages	Disadvantages	Comment
			No cold freon effect	use in an acute attack Must be loaded up correctly	
Diskhaler	30–40 litres/minute	11%	Portable Can carry several doses No cold freon effect	Fiddly May cause bronchoconstriction from powder	Easy for use in children from about five years onwards
Accuhaler	30–90 litres/minute		Dose counter portable	Possible effect of powder causing bronchoconstriction	Easy for use in children from about five years onwards
Turbohaler	30–60 litres/minute	17–32%	Portable Easy for young and the elderly to use	Must not be breathed into as can cause the powder to clog	Needs to be loaded at not less than 45° from vertical or the total dose may be compromised*** May need dose adjustment as with a good technique it is very effective and may have higher absorption
Clickhaler	15–60 litres/minute	29.8%	Portable Dose Counter	Effective at low inspiratory flow rates	

Source: *Barry and O'Callaghan, 1996, **O'Callaghan et al., 1993, ***Prahl and Jensen, 1987 and Brow et al., 1990.

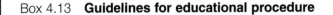

Box 4.13 **Guidelines for educational procedure**

- Demonstrate the appropriate devices
- Supervised practice
- Device selection
- Reading of the accompanying patient instruction leaflet
- Practice with selected device
- Advice on after care of device and cleaning instructions
- Literature to back up technique to take home

Source: Adapted from Linda Pearce NT KNOWHOW, 1998.

Breath Actuated Devices

Patient inhaling activates these devices, which contains a vacuum operated trigger mechanism with the drug being propelled from the canister by CFC propellants. Although, like all pMDIs, they will gradually be replaced by CFC-free propellants. They are in general easier to use than metered dose inhalers, because they do not require the same degree of co-ordination. They are suitable for use from around 6 years of age. As with any inhaler it is important to teach the technique thoroughly, especially as some breath actuated inhalers produce a click on inspiration that may interrupt full inhalation.

Dry Powder Devices

First introduced as single dose devices, the newer devices come as multi-dose versions for use with a range of therapies. Many of them have a dose counter or warning indicator if it is running out. The technique for using them differs from metered dose inhalers, as they require faster and deeper inspiration. The inspiratory effort required for good deposition varies from device to device but is usually between 30 and 60 litres. The devices are breath actuated which again simplifies the use and teaching of them. The powder is held in a reservoir with a built in resistance, so that when the patient inhales the powder is agitated and broken down into respirable particles of varying sizes. It is this internal resistance that dictates the degree of respiratory effort needed to successfully get enough of the drug to the lower airways.

The powder or lactose carriers can act as irritants causing coughing or wheezing in some patients, just as aerosols can in others. It is important not to exhale through the device as it may cause clogging. Dry powder devices are not considered suitable for patients on high dose inhaled steroids as the risk of local and systemic side effects is increased. Patients using over 800 mcgs daily should use metered dose inhalers and a spacer device (BTS Guidelines, 1997).

Assessing Inspiratory Rate

Until recently there was no device available to measure the resistance of dry powder devices. However, recently an inhaler assessment device, the In-Check, has been designed to provide an objective measurement of optimum inspiratory flow of the various inhalers (see Figure 4.5). Devices have varying degrees of inspiratory flow resistance ranging from very little resistance in breath actuated devices to a much greater degree in breath operated devices such as the Turbohaler. It is resistance in some devices that causes the aggregation that enables particles to be broken down into respirable fractions, that is between 2 and 5 μm. If the desired inspiratory flow is not achieved then the fine particle fraction may be considerably reduced, thereby possibly having an effect on asthma control.

While the device is very new, it may, in the future, prove to be very useful for the following:

- preliminary assessments as an aid to choosing the correct device to match the patients inspiratory flow rate

- in routine follow up to check the flow rate remains correct

- to assess whether poor asthma control is possibly due to a basic inability to get a therapeutic dose to the airways

- in more acute asthma, to ensure that a sufficient amount of the dose is reaching the airway

The results obtained are checked against a minimum flow and optimum flow chart (see Table 4.5). As demonstrated above, it is important not to apply conclusions from one inhaler to another of the same class. When changing devices each drug and its dosage should be considered afresh.

Figure 4.5 In-check kit

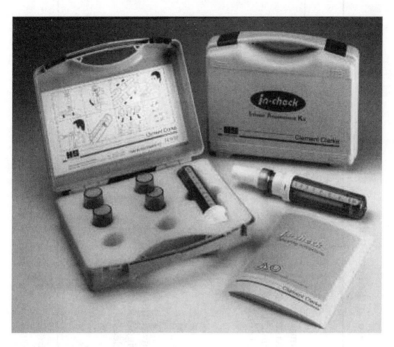

Source: By kind permission of Clement Clarke

Spacers

Spacers are holding devices that enable the patient to breathe in medication from aerosols without the need to co-ordinate actuating the device as well as breathing in properly. If used properly this results in greater deposition of medication to the airways. Other advantages to using a spacer are that there is lower oropharyngeal deposition because the large particles are maintained in the spacer. Therefore, the potential for developing the side effects oral thrush and dysphonia are minimised. This is particularly important for patients requiring high does of inhaled steroids.

Spacers are the best way to deliver medication to children aged under four. However, for small babies large volume spacers with masks may be difficult to use because of the dead space of 50 ml between valve and mask and the effort required to move the drug from the spacer. We need also to take into account, the 'unscientific facts' of acceptability to the patient and carer, and that, in a small baby, a large volume spacer must seem both gigantic and terrifying. The leaflet reproduced in the Appendix A4.1 addresses the problems of using spacers with babies and toddlers.

Table 4.5 In-check minimum and optimum inspiratory flows

DPI Devices ID	Adapter ID	Minimum Flow	Optimum Flow	Variation in dose over range
		Manufacturer's recommended minimum flow rate (L/min)	Flow rate at which optimum dose observed (L/min)	
Turbulent flow inhaler	T	30	60	High
Multiple-dose powder inhaler	A/A/D	30	30	Low
Aerosol capsule inhaler	F	60	120	High
Breath actuated MDIs		Flow required to trigger medication release (L/min)	Flow rate at which optimum dose observed (L/min)	
Auto inhaler	A/A/D	30	30	v. Low
Breath-Actuated inhaler	E/S	20	20	N/A

Source: Adapted from In-Check Inhaler Assessment Kit (© 1998 Clement Clarke International Limited).

Iles *et al.* (1999) have shown that a crying child does not inhale properly, thereby significantly reducing absorption of the aerosolised drugs, so it is not correct to assume that a distressed child has received an adequate dose. Research indicates that particles settle in the spacer within a few seconds (Barry *et al.*, 1993; O'Callaghan *et al.*, 1993). When using small volume spacers there is evidence to show that with small lung volume a few small breaths from a small spacer may result in a greater quantity of drug reaching the airways (Everard *et al.*, 1992). This is particularly so in tidal volumes under 50 ml. Over 150 ml the advantage is lost, therefore, older children may derive greater benefit from larger volume spacers. The Babyhaler has a 350 ml volume and can be used up to school age children, or a Volumatic or Nebuhaler, which both have volumes of 750 ml.

Time, patience and consistency in approach to delivery are what is required for successful management of inhaler devices in the very young. The use of spacer devices should be encouraged when using high doses of inhaled steroids to reduce oral deposition and the possibility of local

---

Box 4.14 **NEBULISERS**

Advantages	Disadvantages
Delivers high dose of drug	Expensive upkeep
Useful in acute situation	Expensive for drugs
Useful in cystic fibrosis for antibiotic inhaled therapy	Not portable
	Needs servicing
Some use in COPD patients	Management for general practice includes using once only products properly i.e. disposable masks and tubing and being responsible for regular servicing.
Must have compatible nebuliser and compressor units	
Face masks must be held on the face or the percentage drug deposition falls markedly	
	Over-use may mask symptoms in acute asthma
Using mouthpieces increases the percentage of drug reaching the airways	Time consuming
	Drug deposition is dependent on the output from the nebuliser and the tidal volume of the patient
	Nebulised ipratroprium may cause acute angle glaucoma in adults and should therefore be used with a mouthpiece
	Low percentage of drug in chamber reaches the patient

and systemic side effects. Compliance with spacers is not always good, therefore, careful explanation of the benefits must be given to the patient or carer.

Nebulisers

Nebulisers are devices that deliver large quantities of drug over a longer period of time than other inhalers, at around ten minutes depending on the type of nebuliser, its efficiency and the drugs used. They have both advantages and disadvantages (see Box 4.14).

Conclusion

It is clear that asthma is a complex inflammatory disease process with a variety of symptoms, problems with diagnosis, multiple treatments and modes of delivery. It therefore requires a structured approach to assessment and management as highlighted. The next chapter examines acute asthma and asthma management within the framework of the BTS guidelines (1997).

Appendix

A4.1 How to use spacers with babies and toddlers

Information for parents

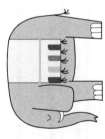

1. Helping an infant use a spacer and mask to treat chest problems

You have just been given a spacer, mask and inhaler to treat your child's chest problems. Whilst you are keen to get on with the prescribed treatment, it is important that your child is happy with the device... so do not rush in, pin your child down with a mask over their face and expect them to be happy with you!

2. Why give medication like this?

Because you can give a smaller dose directly to the lungs where the disease is. This will help reduce the possible side effects than medication taken by mouth.

3. So what is there to do?

First of all unpack the spacer, mask and inhaler and make sure they all fit together. Read the instructions which are in all the boxes.

The spacer has a valve in it which opens when your child breathes in and closes when your child breathes out. The valve on the Volumatic and Nebuhaler make a clicking sound when the valve moves. The Aerochamber and Babyhaler do not make any noise.

4. How to help your child get used to the mask & spacer:

◊ Over the next day or so introduce the mask and spacer to your child

◊ Put your child in a highchair or pushchair so they can see your face (& not make an escape bid!) and let them hold the mask, feel it, touch it and even chew it!

◊ We recommend you play some counting games during which time your child will get used to the mask over their nose and mouth for a longer and longer period of time

◊ Gradually place the mask attached to the spacer over their face. In playing with them *count out loud* very quickly from 1–5, *then take the mask off their face*

◊ Repeat this about ten times then put the mask, spacer & inhaler away

◊ Repeat this regularly throughout the day. Gradually if your child is happy, slow down the counting so that each of your counts corresponds with each of your child's breaths

◊ At the end of the count to five you *must always take the mask off your child's face* as they are learning to associate the end of the count to five with the mask being taken off their face

◊ Gradually over time they will let you keep the mask on their face for five of their breaths without any problems - but make sure you always count out loud as they can't count in their heads!

5. How to use the mask and spacer when your child is used to the mask

◊ Put the mask and spacer together

◊ Shake the inhaler and put into the end of the spacer

◊ Hold the spacer horizontally with the mask over your child's face

◊ Press the inhaler *once* and let your child breathe five times as you count

◊ You should be able to hear the clicking sound with the Volumatic and Nebuhaler—one click for each breath

◊ If you have to give another puff of the medication shake the inhaler and repeat as above

◊ Wash your child's face if they are having inhaled steroids to remove any droplets from the skin

6. No clicking sound when using the Volumatic or Nebuhaler?

◊ If your child is very young they may not be able to breathe hard enough to make the valve move and click

◊ In this case you should hold the spacer and mask at 45° angle to your child's face which will open the valve and the medication will go through the mask with the force of the inhaler and your child's breathing

◊ When your child is in bed you could tip the spacer straight upwards but do not split the spacer open and use like an open cup

7. You must *never, ever* squirt the inhaler straight into a young child's mouth. A child cannot co-ordinate the action of using an inhaler without a spacer device until they are about 11-12 years old. If you do squirt the inhaler directly into their mouth the y will get a sore mouth, unwanted side effects and no benefit from the medication. At about the age of five they may be able to start using a breath activated device such as the Accuhaler, Autohaler, Diskhaler, Turbohaler or Easibreathe.

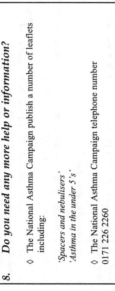

8. Do you need any more help or information?

◊ The National Asthma Campaign publish a number of leaflets including:

  'Spacers and nebulisers'
  'Asthma in the under 5's'

◊ The National Asthma Campaign telephone number
   0171 226 2260

◊ The National Asthma Campaign Helpline number
   0345 01 02 03

◊ Ask your asthma nurse either in hospital or at the GP surgery

◊ Ask other parents how they have managed

© Produced by Jenny Pool, Clinical Nurse Specialist in Childhood Asthma, Addenbrookes NHS Trust. Supported by 3M.

5

Asthma Management

ALISON PARKER

Asthma Never Kills (Salter, 1860)

The above quote from the 19th century is no longer true, as the chart from the National Asthma Campaign (NAC) shows (see Box 5.1). Over recent years the death rate has begun to decline, due to better management, increased use of inhaled steroids and impetus from primary care nurse run asthma clinics (Dickinson *et al.*, 1997; Hoskins, 1998). Salter's remedies including tobacco smoking, morphine and cold baths have not been clinically proven to alleviate or prevent the symptoms of asthma. Even now, nearly a century and-a-half later, there remains debate over the best way in which to treat asthma and prevent asthma deaths, 80 per cent of which are potentially preventable, given better management and education (British Thoracic Association, 1992).

This chapter aims to look at the management of acute asthma and its particular needs, via assessments of what went wrong and how to prevent

---

Box 5.1 **Deaths with asthma registered as the principal cause**

Number of Deaths

	1997	1996	1995	1994	1993	1992
England & Wales	1439	1349	1459	1516	1701	1791
Scotland	113	122	120	119	120	115
N Ireland	32	31	42	30	58	53
UK total	1584	1502	1621	1665	1879	1959

Source: National Asthma Audit NAC, 1999/2000 reproduced with permission of National Asthma Campaign

---

further episodes while relating findings to current thinking via research and agreed guidelines of care.

Asthma Management

The aims of asthma management are summarised in Chapter 4. However achieving them is not always easy due to the changing disease profile, effect of triggers, compliance and many other factors.

Emma – A Case Study

This case study follows the management of a child brought from school to a surgery where no doctor is present and the practice nurse initially has to deal with the situation. The aim here is to highlight how to deal safely with this situation using a protocol with an agreed, legal management structure.

You are on your own in the surgery when the receptionist informs you that a ten-year-old child, Emma, has been brought in by a teacher from the local primary school with acute asthma. The following plan outlines the prompts and responses the nurse would follow.

Approach to the Situation

Quickly and calmly with plenty of reassurance and prompt assessment of the need for help, either from the GP, or via a 999 call for an ambulance with paramedics.

Initial Assessment of Emma and Information Required at this Stage?

Establish that she is a known asthmatic either from the notes or from the child. Ensure she has not inhaled a foreign body or is having an anaphylactic reaction to any substance. Observe colour, level of anxiety and whether she is using accessory muscles of respiration. Any cyanotic feature is very rare and indicates life-threatening asthma. Measure her PEFR: identify her known best or predicted PEFR for height and what is the percentage of this reading to it. If a recent PEFR is available, it is best to measure against this as it may be above or below the predicted value for her height and will, therefore, give a more accurate assessment of the severity of this attack.

A peak flow >50%, predicted or best, indicates uncontrolled asthma

A peak flow ⩽ 50% of predicted or best indicates severe asthma

A peak flow of <33% of predicted or best indicates life threatening asthma

Take and record pulse rate.

A pulse rate >140 beats/min in children under five, a pulse rate of >120 beats/min in 5–15 year olds and a rate of >110 in adults indicates severe asthma

Take and record respiratory rate.

A respiratory rate of >50 breaths per minute in children under 5, a respiratory rate of >40 breaths per minute in 5–15 year olds and a rate of >25 breaths per minute in adults indicates severe asthma

Use of Questioning

To establish the previous use of a bronchodilator and what effect it has had, as well as the duration of symptoms, employ the use of closed questions to the child. Acute asthma is very tiring and being unable to complete sentences is a sign of severe asthma. Some open questions, that is those that require a more detailed answer, can be addressed to the teacher, for example how often has Emma used her reliever this morning?

The Initial Assessment Identifies the Following Information

PEFR 160; Usual Best 310
Pulse Rate 104
Respiratory Rate 24

Emma has an audible wheeze and is using accessory muscles. She is not cyanosed and is able to answer simple questions. In keeping with the BTS Guidelines (1997) for the management of acute severe asthma in general practice you must identify that Emma has uncontrolled asthma and though acute has not at this stage any life threatening features.

In the event that medical aid has not arrived the following treatment would be commenced. First, you should stay with Emma. Either administer salbutamol 5 mgs via a nebuliser *or* give 10 to 20 sequential puffs, singly, through a spacer device. In infants it may be preferable to use a spacer device with a mask as nebulisation may cause paradoxical bronchospasm (British Guidelines on Asthma Management, 1997).

Assess Effectiveness of Treatment

Make an objective assessment: after 15 minutes the PEFR should have increased to at least 75 per cent of best or predicted; the respiratory and pulse rate should both have fallen, although the effect of large doses of β_2 drugs can be to increase the pulse rate; and the use of accessory muscles should be less.

Subjective assessment has established that, Emma feels better, has less cough and/or wheeze and her chest feels less tight. In this instance the nebulised salbutamol has worked well and Emma's peak flow rate is now 270, which is more than 75 per cent of normal; pulse and respiratory rates have also fallen accordingly. The GP has now arrived and has prescribed 30 mgs prednisolone to be taken daily for the next three to five days.

The GP has arranged to see her the next day but what other information would you like to know about her asthma control and treatment?

Current treatment

- what is she currently taking in the way of preventative therapy
- How much reliever is she using
- Compliance: has she been taking the prescribed medication regularly
- Inhaler technique: can she use it correctly, if not reteach or change the device
- Recent symptoms: has she been waking at night coughing or wheezing
- Has she had any day time symptoms and exercise intolerance
- Environment: are there any smokers at home either herself or another household member or visitor
- Are there any new pets at home or at school
- Medication: has she taken any new medication or cold remedy that may contain aspirin or a non-steroidal anti-inflammatory drug, which could have precipitated the acute asthma

Information to give her and her parents before she leaves?

- Reinforce prescription
- Provide information about the preventer, what it is, how and when to take it, the use of oral steroids, advise taking once a day, the reliever and how often she can take it
- Monitoring peak flow; explain what is an acceptable level, how often she should do it and when to seek help if the rate is falling or in conjunction with increasing symptoms

---

Box 5.2 **Aims of acute asthma management**

- Prevent death
- Restore clinical condition and lung function to normal as quickly as possible
- To maintain optimal levels of lung function and health

- It is very important to write the information down and tell her parents and/or teacher
- Arrange review

Throughout this episode the approach is that of support and guidance both physically and psychologically, moving into an educational role as the patient progresses from being acutely ill through to recovery. The principle aims of acute asthma management are summarised in Box 5.2.

Follow up

Thorough follow up is an extremely important aspect following an acute attack or exacerbation. This follow up should be undertaken within 24 hours after an exacerbation and also at the end of the prescribed course of prednisolone. It is important to ensure the patient is back to their best, not requiring a lot of reliever medication and not continuing to have night time wakening due to symptoms. Failure to do this results in suboptimal control, which can lead to long spells of asthma symptoms, as the underlying inflammation has not been adequately suppressed. This is due to the stage three, late phase where exposure to an allergen produces mediators, which cause a smooth muscle contraction within three minutes, and usually subsides within 30 to 60 minutes. A late phase response may occur between four to eight hours later (Holgate, 1996). This is due to an influx of eosonophils and neutrophils in to the area, which increases the bronchial responsiveness and airway obstruction due to increased inflammatory processes. This late phase may last from days to several weeks, which then predispose the patient to further acute exacerbations, and might put them at risk of developing more severe or even fatal asthma (Mohan *et al.*, 1996). An enquiry conducted in East Anglia indicate certain risk factors which need to be considered when assessing and managing acute asthma (see Box 5.3).

Box 5.3   **Patients at risk of developing severe or fatal asthma**

Are those:

- with psychiatric morbidity, behavioural difficulties especially denial and socio-economic deprivation; recognise denial by non-attendance, non-compliance with therapy or monitoring, unwillingness to accept the diagnosis or regular therapy

- ever admitted to hospital with their asthma

- requiring emergency steroids and/or nebulisation

- calling GP or attending surgery or A and E department with emergency deterioration

- requiring courses of, or regular, steroids

- requiring high dose inhaled steroids

- whose peak flow falls below 50% of their best or predicted value

- requiring two or more bronchodilator inhalers monthly

Discuss these issues frankly with the patient and their relatives

Source: Mohan *et al.* 'A confidential enquiry into deaths caused by Asthma in an English Health Region: Implications for General Practice', *British Journal General Practice* (1996) 46: 29–32.

A good management strategy would be to agree a plan of care with the patient or carer. Plans are available from the National Asthma Campaign (see Figure A5.1), or you can devise your own. However the most important considerations should be: if known, what are the patients own best peak flow?; at what percentage do they experience more severe asthma? According to Charlton *et al.*, (1990), the key to effective asthma management lies in teaching the patient the importance of their symptoms and the appropriate action to take when their asthma deteriorates. Therefore, in conjunction with peak flow measurement, agree what degree of symptoms and reliever therapy are acceptable, when should they intervene with an increase or decrease in therapy and what action to take if there is no improvement.

This is, therefore, an individual plan taking into consideration all of the above along with known trigger factors and the patients ability or confidence in utilizing it. Often the simpler it is the better. For those people not able to cope with such a plan, drawing a line in red ink under the point on a peak flow chart where they need to seek further help may be an effective form of simple management. It is also important to involve another family member or close friend in the education and management of such patients.

Ongoing Management

Emma was reviewed the following day when it was found that her peak
flow was between 75 and 85 per cent of her best and she was able to sleep.
She was advised to continue the prednisolone for the next three days and
to use salbutamol two puffs, four times a day for the next two days and
then if stable continue to use on an 'as required basis'. An appointment
was made to review her at the end of the steroid course.

She presents now with her mother. Her peak flow is back to her normal
best of 290 l/min in the morning to 310 l/min in the evening. Your assessment today looks at six main factors: night time and day time symptoms,
activity problems, inhaler technique, compliance with medication, peak
flow and what percentage of her normal best it is. Based on the findings
you advise that there is no need for further oral steroids because her peak
flow is greater than 80 per cent of her known best and that her symptom
scoring is now very low.

You now have the opportunity to try to identify what went wrong and
whether this acute attack may have been avoided or dealt with more
efficiently. Should she continue on the double dose of inhaled steroid for a
further week and then, if stable, reduce to her maintenance dose? This
depends on your assessment of what the previous dose was and whether
it was sufficient. You identify from the notes that Emma had been
prescribed fluticasone 50 mcg twice daily via an accuhaler and salbutamol
200 mcg accuhaler one dose when required. According to mum and backed
up by the repeat prescriptions this has been on a very occasional basis.

Compliance

A good starting point may be to ascertain how good the compliance was
with the preventer. The Royal Pharmaceutical Society 1996 describes
non-compliers as being of two distinct categories: intentional and non-
intentional. You might ask 'before your asthma attack last week how often
were you using your preventer inhaler'. However, you might get a more
accurate answer if you ask 'how often do you normally forget to use your
inhaler in a week'. This latter approach acknowledges that people do
forget, that is unintentional non-compliance and reduces their
embarrassment at admitting to forgetting.

It may be, however, that they are intentional non-compliers and that by
careful approach you can establish why. If the non-compliance was
because Emma was so well that they decided to stop the treatment or due
to experiencing few symptoms, she was simply forgetting, then this serves
as a perfect introduction to reinforce education. Discussion centres on the

inflammatory nature of asthma and how it is reduced by regular use of a preventer, reaching an agreement on the treatment pathway between the healthcare team and family. Vathenen *et al.* (1991) showed that adults treated with budesonide for six weeks significantly reduced their airway responsiveness. However, within one week of stopping treatment their symptoms had returned.

If this is deliberate non-compliance then the reason has to be ascertained. Use of open questioning for example 'Some people have worries about using inhaled steroids. How do you feel about this?' should provide a forum for discussing their possible misconceptions of side effects or addiction. It is important that this is taken seriously and that the person dealing with it has enough knowledge to allay such fears. If this is not addressed properly then confidence in the use of the drugs and of the educator will not be gained. This confidence is a very important aspect in building a relationship with the patient and family. To uphold this it is important that the whole asthma team is giving the same message and that treatment pathways are discussed, respected and agreed in practice protocol.

Safety of Drugs

How do you deal with the aspect of safety in drugs? Growth in children is a particular issue of concern and can be addressed by a consistent approach to monitoring. Asthmatic children should have their height and weight recorded on a centile chart biannually (see Box 5.4).

Proper measurement is crucial and should be carried out as outlined in Fry (1998), while serial measurements indicate whether a child is growing normally (Kelnar, 1996). Children whose growth drops by a centile or more should be referred to an endocrinologist, first, having had their treatment

---

Box 5.4   **Height measurement in children**

1. Remove shoes, socks and headwear.
2. Stand feet together with heels touching the back of the vertical plane, legs straight with bottom and shoulder blades touching the vertical plane.
3. Place the measuring arm on the child's head.
4. Ensure the child is looking directly ahead.
5. Read the height to the nearest millimetre.

reviewed. Detrimental effects on growth are not seen in doses of inhaled steroids under 400 mcg daily (Agertoft and Pederson, 1994), however some children may be more sensitive to the effects than others and each has to be assessed individually. There is evidence to show that doses of greater than 400 mcg of beclamethasone may affect short-term growth but the effect on final height is not yet known (Wolthers and Pederson, 1993). A four-year study undertaken in primary care in Tayside found that the majority of children prescribed on inhaled steroids were not affected either in height or in weight (McCowan *et al.*, 1998). However, if they were on step 4 of the treatment guidelines (BTS, 1997) and were receiving shared primary/secondary care they experienced a significant reduction in their stature. They also found that social deprivation had an adverse effect on growth irrespective of any disease process.

Therefore, children who are receiving high doses of inhaled steroids – over 800 mcgs of beclamethasone or budesonide, or over 500 mcgs of fluticasone – should have their growth measured three-monthly and should be under regular review by a paediatrician with a special interest in asthma (Fry, 1998; BTS, 1997). Consideration must also be given to the effects of uncontrolled asthma on growth and the risk–benefit ratio considered.

Symptom Control

The Impact of Asthma survey (NAC, 1996) found 27 per cent of respondents reporting that asthma had a huge impact on their life and 43 per cent having a moderate impact, with a large proportion still experiencing symptoms (see Box 5.5). Therefore, although the knowledge and potential for reducing asthma morbidity with effective treatment exists, there is a deficit either in terms of compliance or in the provision of care from the health care professionals. There are three main issues to consider if you suspect a patient of having symptoms, once compliance has been established:

- is the drug getting to the correct place?
- is the dose correct?
- are they receiving the correct drugs?

We shall consider each in turn. A study by Crompton (1982) found that of 1000 patients known to have been able to use a metered dose inhaler, at follow up 13 per cent had lost the ability. What does this mean in terms of on going education? Because people develop bad habits very quickly, in every asthma review visit the health professional should check the inhaler technique, regardless of any previously known ability of use.

Box 5.5 **Key findings from the Impact of Asthma survey**

- Over one in four respondents (27%) felt that asthma totally controlled their life or had a major effect upon it.

- Over four in ten respondents (42%) felt they experienced asthma symptoms every day or on most days.

- Over four in ten respondents (44%) were woken at night at least once a week by a cough, wheeze or breathlessness.

- In the last year, nearly one in three schoolchildren (32%) were absent for at least one week from school because of asthma.

- Of all respondents aged between 12 and 17 years 81% felt that exercise/activity had at least a moderate effect on their lives.

- Nearly half of all respondents (47%) said they would like more information about asthma.

- More than one in ten respondents (13%) visited a hospital accident and emergency department in the last twelve months because of a severe asthma attack.

Source: NAC, 1996, reproduced with permission.

The delivery of the drug may also be important with some devices delivering a higher dose, so the dosage may need to be altered if a change of device is made. The safest way to use inhaled steroids is via a spacer device thereby maximising the effectiveness, without increasing the dosage, and minimising the side effects (North of England Asthma Guideline Development Group, 1996). However, for smaller doses and to aid compliance, it is essential to agree with the patient the correct device for individual.

If the inhaler technique is correct and compliance is deemed to be good then the next step is to look at the dosage of the preventer. This should be correlated with the objective measurement of serial peak flow readings along with more subjective reporting of symptoms and use of a bronchodilator. However, dosage of the preventer is not now the only consideration in asthma management. Since the initial introduction of the BTS Guidelines in 1993, the management of asthma may appear to have become more complicated, due to a number of factors. There has been a move away from simply increasing the dose of inhaled steroid, to gain control. This is due to:

- there being more evidence regarding the dose response curve of inhaled steroids and concern over safety of high doses, summarised in Lipworth (1999)

- studies which show that the addition of a long acting β_2-agonist to a low dose of inhaled steroids works as well, if not better, than using a high dose of inhaled steroid alone in terms of fewer symptoms and improved lung function (Greening *et al.*, 1994; Woolcock *et al.*, 1996)

- studies which show that the addition of a long acting β_2-agonist reduces acute exacerbations and, therefore, the need for oral steroids, improves lung function and reduces symptoms (Pauwels *et al.*, 1997; Van der Molen *et al.*, 1996).

- a new class of drug to be used at step three in the form of leukotriene modifiers. However, this new class of drugs is still in its infancy and there is less data on how or for whom they will make a difference. Obviously more studies are required. In the meantime there are certain factors as described by Partridge (1998) to consider when making a choice

- patient choice

- cost (to the State or individual)

- potential adverse effect of compliance of multiple regimens

- the potential risks of high dose inhaled steroids

- preference for tablet therapy

- fear of possible systemic side effects.

It is known that there are different subgroups of asthma and as more information becomes available from the results of long-term trials then perhaps these decisions will become easier. Meanwhile, when starting a patient on any new therapy the most important factor is the follow up. It is known that there is a subset of asthmatics for whom long acting β_2-agonists have no effect. According to Kuitert (1999) there is some evidence to suggest that in primary care the anti-leukotriene drugs are beneficial in about 50 per cent of patients. It is important that for those who receive no benefit that the drug is stopped after a trial period and alternatives tried.

The other maxim is to start high then reduce the dose when you gain control. Again it is important that the drug is reduced or the regimen is altered if control is not gained, to avoid patients staying on high doses too long.

Education

Education should be patient focused. The British Lung Foundation defines three main areas for addressing the issues around patient education

- What does the patient want to achieve? This may be quite different to what you think they need.

- What are the barriers to achieving this that is, the patients individual concerns.

- What does the patient already know about asthma?

Self Management

The philosophy of self management is what most people with chronic disease strive for as it empowers them and gives control over their lives. The concept of self management for asthma patients can only be realized in the presence of sufficient information and understanding on the part of the patient or carer. Therefore, the health professional must endeavour to educate the patient on the different aspects of asthma to include:

- the disease process

- their own best lung function

- their own trigger factors

- education re. drugs; their action and how and when to use them

- what action to take when their asthma is worsening.

The principle of self management is that the patient should intervene in the event of worsening asthma to prevent further decline in control and/or to seek help from health care professionals if this has not been successful. There is some debate as to whether it is correct to double inhaled steroids. The BTS Guidelines (1997) acknowledge that there is little evidence to support this strategy. However in the absence of studies it is deemed reasonable to increase dosage, certainly in adults. In children, there have been studies to suggest that doubling the dose of inhaled steroids does not work (Garrett *et al.*, 1998). Although doing so, reinforces the ethos of reducing the inflammation and the need for regular dosage. It is important to ensure that the dose is reduced after the exacerbation. Also, if there has not been a good response to oral steroids or if they need to be continued for longer, a review of the diagnosis is required and a referral to a chest physician if there is any doubt.

If Emma was on a suitable dose with good compliance and good inhaler technique, then either the treatment level was inadequate or she had been ignoring symptoms. Most people with acute asthma do not have sudden onset or brittle asthma. In the majority of patients there has been an increase in symptoms prior to the attack, which have not been dealt with (Rees and Price, 1995).

Environment

Commonly asked questions relate to the environment including air pollution and common allergens such as pets and grasses. The role of air pollution in asthma is controversial and while it has not been linked to developing the disease it has a significant contributory effect on the health and subsequent increased symptoms and drug treatment in children and adults (Burr, 1995; Gielen *et al.*, 1997; Nicolai, 1999).

However, the indoor environment is probably more relevant, with the changes in lifestyle over the last generation possibly accounting in part for the rising incidence of asthma and atopy. Approximately 80 per cent of asthmatic children are allergic to house dust mite and pets (Warner *et al.*, 1978). In the UK over 50 per cent of homes have either a cat or dog (Warner *et al.*, 1991) and, therefore, the implementation of avoidance measures and allergen reduction is made difficult.

Whether one is skin prick tested to allergens or not depends to a degree on the availability of the service and on the history obtained from the patient. The results have to be seen in context to the symptomatology and degree of morbidity experienced by the patient, with specific advice then tailored to them. The avoidance of provoking factors where possible (BTS, 1997) should be in conjunction with or complementary to drug treatment (Cross *et al.*, 1998). For example inhaled corticosteroids in asthma along with avoidance measures for house dust mite or allergen (see Box 5.6 and Box 5.7).

It is important to treat the concurrent symptoms of seasonal or perennial rhinitis as often asthma control improves. The nose is primarily a filter. If someone is unable to breathe through it then they breathe a much higher concentration of allergens directly into the lungs through their

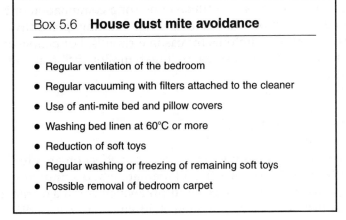

Box 5.6 **House dust mite avoidance**

- Regular ventilation of the bedroom
- Regular vacuuming with filters attached to the cleaner
- Use of anti-mite bed and pillow covers
- Washing bed linen at 60°C or more
- Reduction of soft toys
- Regular washing or freezing of remaining soft toys
- Possible removal of bedroom carpet

Box 5.7   **Reduction of animal allergens**

- Keep furry pets outdoors
- Not cleaning the cages of small animals
- Bathing the pet weekly to reduce allergen
- Removing the bedroom carpet

NB Removing pets and employing subsequent cleaning measures can still take six months to reduce the level of allergens in the home.

Box 5.8   **Pollen in hay fever**

- Close windows especially at night
- Wear sunglasses
- Have a pollen filter in the car
- Avoid walking in grassy areas
- Start preventive treatment in advance of known worst season

mouth, thereby increasing the inflammatory process and subsequently the asthma symptoms. If it is mainly the nose that is affected then treatment with topical corticosteroids to control symptoms should suffice. However if the eyes are affected then antihistamines or a combination of both may be required. Education should encourage starting preventive therapy prior to the onset of symptoms in seasonal rhinitis. For people with more severe hay fever the measures outlined in Box 5.8 may need to be employed.

Smoking – Adult and Child

Both active and passive smoking has a direct effect on an adult's asthma control in terms of increasing the inflammation and symptoms. It is now recognized that maternal smoking in pregnancy is a major risk factor in the development of asthma in young children (Sears *et al.*, 1996).

Conclusion

Asthma care is a complex subject requiring a consistent evidence based and positive approach to management. The space available does not allow in depth discussion of some issues, which are very important, such as occupational asthma in adults, which would need to be addressed in the same systematic way.

Appendix

Figure A 5.1   A plan of care

ASTHMA ACTION PLAN
for tiddlers and toddlers

Child's name   ....

Date   ....

This is an Action Asthma Plan for asthmatic children who cannot do peak flows. This plan will help you adjust your child's treatment according to symptoms.

Usual preventative (brown/orange) treatment: ....

Usual relieving (blue) treatment: ....

Other treatment: ....

Device:

....

Usually the blue reliever should only be given when needed for shortness of breath, coughing, wheezing or before exercise to prevent symptoms.

1. Good control

Your child should be well with no restriction on exercise or other daily activities. They should ı be disturbed by coughing or wheezing at night.

Your child should remain on the usual medication outlined above and not need to take the blue reliever more than twice a day.

2.   Deteriorating control

If your child is waking at night with coughing or wheeze
<u>or</u> is unable to exercise as usual
<u>or</u> is needing blue reliever more than twice a day
<u>or</u> is starting a cold (if this is your child's trigger)

What to do:

- Give blue reliever every four hours
- Double the brown/orange preventer (inhaled steroids)

Carry on with this until your child has been symptom free and well for three to five days. If your child requires regular reliever for more than two or three days <u>without improvement</u> see your GP.

3. Severe attack

Your child is showing poor response to the blue reliever i.e. still has symptoms 30 mins after the reliever is given
<u>or</u> is needing blue reliever again within 2 hours
<u>or</u> is unable to walk, talk or play normally due to breathlessness
<u>or</u> has laboured breathing (or pulling in of the lower ribs and upper tummy)

What to do:

- Give the blue reliever every four hours (this may be by the nebuliser or via the spacer)
- Double the brown/orange inhaled steroids
- See your GP <u>that day</u> for a 3—5 day course of oral steroids.
- <u>or</u> give oral steroids (prednisolone .... mg - .... tablets) once a day for three to five days if this has been discussed with you by your GP or hospital staff. If you do this contact your GP and tell them what you have done and arrange for child to be seen within 24 hours
- when over the acute attack go to step 2 (deteriorating control) and follow this advice!

---

4. Emergency

If your child needs the blue reliever within 30 mins of giving the last dose
<u>or</u> the reliever does not seem to work at all
<u>or</u> your child is blue around lips and tongue
<u>or</u> your child cannot talk or eat due to breathlessness

Help is required urgently.

- Unless a doctor can come immediately then you should take your child immediately to local hospital

- You should call 999 for an ambulance if you do not have transport or are alone with your child

- You should also give treatment every 15 mins whilst awaiting help — either through a spacer or the nebuliser

---

Source: © Jenny Pool, Clinical Nurse Specialist in Childhood Asthma, Children's Services, Addenbrookes Hospital, CAmbrid

Part III

Teamwork in Chronic Disease

6

The Concept of Teamwork

SUE PAULSON

The epidemiology of diabetes illustrates the rationale for effective multidisciplinary teamwork, as this condition impinges on every aspect of the patient's lifestyle. All personnel involved in the management of diabetes need to have the skills to work together effectively. Empowerment of the patient with diabetes emphasizes the need for a team which functions at an optimum level, with good communication skills. Such a team is multidisciplinary, requiring the input of a range of healthcare professionals, such as diabetes specialist nurses, hospital and community nurses, doctors, dieticians, occupational health nurses and chiropodists. Clinical governance especially emphasizes the corporate accountability of healthcare professionals working together as team members because Trust chief executives are now accountable to parliament for delivering quality clinical care. This means that the quality of health service provision has the same weight in statute as financial accountability (Millar, 1999).

The concept of teamwork is complex due to the dynamic interaction of health care professionals with very different roles. There may be several different teams involved in caring for the patient with diabetes, such as a hospital team and a community team, and good communication is needed both within these teams and between these teams. There are many different lines of communication between healthcare professionals themselves and between healthcare professionals and patients. The idea of interactions in teams being circular, involving both positive and negative feedback, comes from systems theory, which studies how families can become locked into certain patterns of interaction. Teams can certainly become locked into particular patterns of circular interaction that function to maintain homeostasis or the status quo. An element of creativity is needed to prevent stagnation from happening (Jones, 1993).

Within a particular healthcare team, it is useful to identify clearly the task and how the different roles of healthcare professionals can contribute to the performance of the task. A written philosophy can be a useful tool for identifying the particular aims of a healthcare team. To be effective, a healthcare team needs to have a balance between the strengths and weaknesses of its individual members. This means the weaknesses in the team should be compensated by the strengths. The result is a 'theory of allowable weaknesses' within a team, which is particularly compensated by strengths, such as the skills of the team leader. When the team leader is a nurse, such as a district nursing sister or diabetic specialist, their strengths lie in role-modelling expert clinical skills to junior nurses and, of course, the individuals with diabetes themselves. The team leader has the responsibility of appropriately delegating the different aspects of care of the person with diabetes, such as producing patient education materials and training and assessment of staff in the use of equipment and clinical procedures.

Barbara Scammell (1990) has particularly emphasized the 'theory of allowable weaknesses' as being pertinent to an effective team. She suggests each team member needs to have a specific role within the team. There should be a clever/creative member who works with the team leader and accepts the team leader's authority. Other team members should show a mixture of abilities but these abilities must be appropriate to their specific roles. The weaknesses in the team should be compensated by the team's overall strengths. For example, it does not matter if one individual member does not want to take on responsibility for formally assessing junior staff, as long as their clinical skills are adequate. Neither does it matter if one individual member does not want to take on responsibility for actually producing patient education materials, as long as their knowledge base is adequate for utilizing any such materials. It is interesting to note that in this theory of allowable weaknesses, Scammell sees the most difficult members as being those whose contribution to the team is regarded as a liability. She also describes how team members who are allocated roles, which they have not chosen or which are inappropriate for them, become bored, anxious, or belligerent.

Case study: Teamwork in a District Nursing Context

A district nursing team comprised one nurse manager, two nursing sisters, six staff nurses, four health care assistants – at varying levels of their training – and two second year nursing students. The strengths of the nurse manager related to organisational and communication skills, especially the dissemination of information among the nursing team and liaison with the multi-disciplinary team as a whole. The weaknesses of the nurse manager related to being overstretched and having too many jobs to do. The strengths of the two nursing sisters related to role-modelling nursing care and acting as a team leader, managing the community workload on a daily basis and providing educational programmes to maintain standards of nursing care. The weaknesses of these two nursing sisters related to having too much to do and lack of time to give feedback and support to junior staff. The strengths of the staff nurses related to the delivery of appropriate nursing care on a daily basis and the ability to support other team members. The weaknesses of these staff nurses related to their lack of depth in clinical knowledge and organizational skills, besides little appreciation of the overall picture of the management of the community workload. The strengths of the health care assistants related to their ability to give hands on care to the patients and their willingness to feedback information. The weaknesses of these healthcare assistants related to their difficulty in appreciating the importance of the trained nurses' roles. The strengths of the student nurses related to their eagerness to learn and an up-to-date basic level of knowledge. The weaknesses of the student nurses related to their lack of ability in applying this basic knowledge to practice.

Activity

Make a chart with three columns, identifying each role with its respective strengths and weaknesses. Which members of the team run the risk of becoming what Barbara Scammell (1990) has described as 'difficult' members? Do you think this district nursing team would function effectively as a whole?

1. Add the following roles to the chart to complete the picture of a multi-disciplinary team and identify their potential strengths and weaknesses: occupational therapist, physiotherapist, social worker, chiropodist, and dietician. Do you think the nursing team in the case study would be able to function effectively as part of the wider multi-disciplinary team?

2. Using a large sheet of paper to jot your ideas on, identify the different roles within the health care team to which you belong. Alongside each role, identify the strengths and weaknesses of that particular role. Share your ideas with a colleague. Evaluate the implications of your particular team's strengths and weaknesses for the functioning of the team as a whole. Does your team complete its work effectively? Remember the theory of allowable weaknesses.

Group Processes are Involved in Teamwork

When convening a completely new healthcare team, the four stages of the theory of group processes can be seen. Burnard (1995) has identified these four stages as: the forming stage; the storming stage; the norming stage; and the performing stage. The first stage in group processes then is the forming stage when group members meet and slowly get to know each other. Minimal trust and self-disclosure is shown at this stage and little in terms of the task is achieved by the group. The second stage in group processes is the storming stage when relationships between members are explored more fully, conflict occurs between group members and there is tension between the needs of the group as a whole and the needs of individual group members. The third stage is the norming stage when the group develops cohesiveness through establishing rules and resolving conflicts. Individual group members who are unhappy with the particular group will have left by this stage. The fourth and final stage in group processes is the performing stage when the group becomes mature and productive, with the group working effectively together while accepting the different strengths and weaknesses of its individual members. The weakness at this last stage is the risk of stagnation or the group thinking as one and losing its potential for creativity.

Within your particular healthcare team, these group processes may not be so clearly identifiable, as individual healthcare professionals may be involved with the team for differing lengths of time. When there are a number of new recruits, the four stages are more obvious as the group has to form a new identity, resolve different conflicts, establish fresh norms or rules, and get down to performing the task.

Activity

1. List the norms or the rules that operate within your healthcare team. For example, one norm could be 'Nursing care must be patient-centred, respecting the wishes of the patient and their family.' Do these norms/rules contribute to the effectiveness of the team as a whole? How did these norms/rules originate in the first instance?

Share your ideas with another member of your healthcare team to see if they have a different perception of which norms/rules operate within the team. Alternatively, share your ideas with a healthcare professional from a different team. Do different norms/rules operate within different healthcare teams? How can you explain the similarities/differences?

Specific Communication Interactions within Group Processes

Within any healthcare team, there may be evidence of certain types of interactions occurring within the group processes. The way these interactions have been described reflects theories of both conscious and unconscious processes occurring. Burnard (1995) has described group processes in conscious terms, but acknowledges the influence of psychodynamic thinking that emphasizes unconscious processes at work within any group. Menzies-Lyth's (1988) model of unconscious processes at work within a healthcare team is considered later in the chapter as an example of how the emotional needs of a group heavily influence how it functions.

Activity

1. Identify the different ways in which you communicate within your nursing team and between your nursing team and the multi-disciplinary team. Brainstorm your ideas on a large sheet of paper. Do you notice both formal and informal ways of communicating within your team? Do the informal ways of communicating sometimes get in the way of the formal work of the team?

You may have found yourself initially listing all the formal ways of communication such as written documentation, word-processing, and telephone/fax. Nursing handovers, case conferences and meetings at GP's surgeries seem to span both formal and informal ways of communication. When interpersonal communication is face to face, it taps into both verbal and non-verbal skills, particularly through the expression of emotion by gossip or humour. There is a sense in which the emotional needs of individual members of the team become entangled with the formal work agenda. How individual members of the team relate to each other takes on a vital significance in the performance of the formal work agenda.

Burnard (1995) describes specific interactions within healthcare teams, which may be identified in any context. These specific interactions can hinder the functioning of the group as a whole.

1. Pairing occurs when two group members talk to each other rather than the group.

2. Projection occurs when group members blame the group for the way they are feeling rather than owning the feeling themselves.

3. Scapegoating occurs when the group takes out their hostile feelings on one member.

4. Shutting down occurs when a group member isolates themselves from the group, often becoming emotionally distraught in the process.

5. Rescuing occurs when a group member defends others from attack.

6. Flight occurs when the group avoids serious issues by humour, intellectualising or changing the subject.

The case study earlier in the text identified strengths and weaknesses in different members of a district nursing team and hinted at the issue of emotionality and stress. The potential of emotionality and stress was implied as the district nursing sisters were overstretched, with too many jobs to do and insufficient time to give feedback to junior nurses. This relates to Burnard's (1995) idea of specific interactions within group processes, which can actually hinder the functioning of the group and so, the performance of the work agenda. There is the implication that the district nursing sisters are actually having to 'shut down' a little in order to cope with their workload which means junior staff are perhaps not getting enough support. This idea of 'shutting down' carries the risk of emotional distress, suggesting the district nurses in this particular case study may be feeling stressed.

Activity

1. Reflect on the healthcare team in which you are involved. Identify specific examples of the interactions in group processes identified by Burnard (1995). For example, two staff nurses on a district nursing team may show 'pairing' behaviour, talking to each other at a case conference rather than to the whole team, or a nurse who is feeling 'overstretched' may project their feelings onto the whole team. Think about interventions you could make to improve communication within your team.

Unconscious Communication in Group Processes

From psychodynamic theory, there is the concept of any group/team of people having both a conscious, task-orientated agenda and an unconscious agenda of emotional needs, which may be in conflict with the needs of the task. Freud in the early 1900s conducted the original psychodynamic study of ego defence mechanisms; unconscious processes that develop in the individual to relieve unconscious anxieties. Such individual unconscious defence mechanisms can be seen at work within any group or team, restricting performance on the conscious task-orientated agenda. Individual unconscious defence mechanisms include repression of threatening thoughts, displacement of feelings onto another person or object because they cannot be shown openly, denial of certain aspects of reality because it is too painful, intellectualisation about behaviour which is unacceptable, identification with another person's perspective and projection of unwanted feelings onto another person. Isolation is an unconscious defence mechanism used by the individual to separate contradictory feelings and regression means the individual goes back to an earlier stage of development (Gross, 1996).

Burnard (1995) has hinted at the role of the unconscious in determining how individuals interact in healthcare teams through the group processes of pairing, projection, scapegoating, shutting down, rescuing and flight outlined earlier in the text. These group processes build on the work of Bion (1961) with traumatised Second World War soldiers who applied the idea of unconscious defence mechanisms to group therapy. Bion (1961) found unconscious group processes – similar to the group processes identified by Burnard (1995) – created a feeling of a group acting as a living organism. Bion's (1961) three basic assumptions of the unconscious processes in groups concern

1. dependency: when the group acts as if it has to find a leader to meet its needs;

2. fight/flight: when the group acts as if it has to attack or flee from an enemy within the group; and

3. pairing: when two group members work together or against each other in order to create a 'saviour' for the group's problems.

This takes group processes much further than simply seeing them in terms of norms and roles with emergent patterns of communication and a conscious task agenda. Bion (1961) introduced the concept of the group functioning as an entity, developing from the idea of individuals having unconscious motivations or emotional needs which influence the conscious and unconscious communication patterns between group members. Bion (1961) especially emphasized the splitting of good and bad emotions within the individual, the projection of emotions from one individual to another within the group and the individual who received the projected emotions then identifying with them. Menzies-Lyth (1988) has developed this idea of the group functioning as a group at the level of emotionality among healthcare professionals.

The Nursing Team Functioning as a Living Organism

Case Study 1: Emotional Involvement

At a sixteen bedded hospice, there was a nursing team comprising 20 members. There was a mixture of staff nurses of varying experience and a large number of health care assistants besides a clinical nurse manager. The atmosphere was relaxed and friendly, the patients were very sick, requiring a lot of nursing care, and their families needed a lot of emotional support. The intensity of the work meant that the nurses were very involved with the patients in their particular team and the smallness of the unit created the feeling that the nurses were very involved with each other. The nurses seemed very wrapped up in each other's lives on an emotional level. This related to Bion's concept of the group functioning as a living organism with unconscious communication occurring through splitting, projection and identification. There was evidence of individual members of staff splitting their good and bad feelings and projecting both their good and bad feelings onto others. One particular member of staff seemed to receive the projections of all the negative emotions from the group and identified with this role.

Activity

Reflect on the reasons for this particular nursing team being so involved with each other on an emotional level. Do you think this helped the team to function on the conscious, work agenda?

Menzies-Lyth (1988) studied the unconscious processes operating in a London teaching hospital and her ideas have been applied to unconscious processes operating in other work organisations (Obholzer and Roberts, 1994). The idea of unconscious processes hindering the conscious task-orientated agenda can be extrapolated to nursing teams in any setting, including the primary healthcare team. The organisation is used by those who work within it to produce social structures that will reduce anxiety. Organisational practices function as institutional defences, collective externalisation's of individual psychological defences. Unconscious defence mechanisms among nursing staff may include:

1. splitting of the nurse–patient relationship
2. depersonalisation, categorisation and denial of the significance of the individual
3. detachment and denial of feelings
4. the attempt to eliminate decisions by ritual task performance
5. collusive social redistribution of responsibility and irresponsibility.

These defence mechanisms, which reduce anxiety, also reduce job satisfaction, depriving nurses of necessary reassurances and preventing them from making personal contributions. Opportunities for conscious reflection or change are minimised within the organisation as a result.

Case Study 2: Defence Mechanisms

A multi-disciplinary team meeting was being held at a GP's surgery to plan care for elderly people with diabetes. There was a discussion about an elderly insulin-dependent diabetic woman who was blind and her husband who was developing Alzheimer's and could no longer help her safely with her injections. The healthcare team used a number of defence mechanisms to cope with this difficult scenario. A number of different healthcare personnel had been involved in caring for the couple. During the course of this discussion, the woman was called the 'diabetic patient' and her husband was called the 'Alzheimer's patient'. Nursing care had focused on management of the woman's diabetes and assessing the safety of the husband. The social worker was instructed to find out about residential care as a matter of urgency.

Activities

1. Identify which defence mechanisms were being used in this case study.

2. Think of a particular scenario within your own healthcare team where defence mechanisms are used. Identify the particular defence mechanisms and suggest ways for supporting your team so that more open communication is possible.

Strategies to Improve Teamwork

Communication Models Pertinent to Teamwork

Heron (1989) provided a useful model of the conscious processes in interpersonal communication, which has been extrapolated to the nursing context by Burnard (1995). See if the interventions you identified to improve communication within your healthcare team relate to any of Heron's Six Category Intervention analysis (1989) outlined below. In simple terms, Heron (1989) identified three categories of intervention/styles of communicating where the nurse uses authority and three categories of intervention/styles of communicating where the nurse takes a facilitative role. Such a model is applicable to nurse–patient relationships besides relationships within the nursing team. It is an interesting model to use for a reflective diary to analyse how relationships develop within a nursing team. While each of the six categories suggests a particular style of communicating within a nursing team, it soon becomes apparent that several styles may be used at once in a specific episode of interpersonal communication. As the model comes from a tradition of humanistic psychology, which sees individual people as conscious of their thought processes and able to exert personal agency or choice, it recognizes the right of the other person to refuse the communication request. This means the communication request may need to be repeated, potentially in a different style or from a different person within the health care team.

Outline of Heron's Six Category Intervention Analysis as a Communication Model (1989)

Authoritative Interventions

1. *Prescriptive interventions*: recommend and evaluate behaviour to the other person, so enhancing their self-determination. Such interventions are necessary in a medical emergency

2. *Informative interventions*: give information and interpret behaviour to the other person, enhancing independent thinking and self-awareness.

3. *Confronting interventions:* challenge the attitudes and behaviours of the other person, enhancing their self awareness. Such interventions highlight difficult points and need to be well timed and respectful of the other person, using a clear, calm, and supportive approach. There should be no aggression and no 'pussyfooting' or skirting around the issue.

Facilitative Interventions

4. *Supportive interventions*: affirm the value of the other person through unconditional positive regard, using listening skills. Solidarity is shown through non-verbal communication, such as touch and facial expression. Discreet self-disclosure may be used for the benefit of the other person. Selective reflection, repeating the other person's last few words or emotionally charged words, encourages the other person to explore ideas.

5. *Catalytic interventions*: elicit information from the other person through using open questions for self discovery and closed questions for exploring specific areas. The other person is invited to change through self generated insight and support from active listening and selective reflection.

6. *Cathartic interventions*: release tensions through laughter, crying, or anger. Such interventions should be at a level of distress the other person

can handle and the other person needs time to reflect on the experience of catharsis, identifying any new insights.

Activities

1. Classify all the different ways of communicating within the healthcare team, which you identified in the previous activity under the appropriate category or categories of Heron's Six Category Intervention analysis. Do you see overlaps between the authoritative and facilitative categories of intervention? What are the implications of such overlaps for communication within your healthcare team?

2. Plan a teaching session on the care of diabetic patients for your primary health care team, using selected material from the following two chapters of this book and Heron's Six Category Intervention Analysis as a framework. Balance facilitative and authoritative interventions, for example, the session could be started with a catalytic intervention, using open and closed questions to assess your team's existing level of knowledge, utilize a supportive intervention to highlight relevant contributions and a confronting intervention to challenge misconceptions, supplemented by an informative intervention.

3. Focus on the *confronting* category in Heron's Six Category Intervention Analysis. Burnard (1995) suggests this is one of the categories nurses find most difficult to use. Think of a situation where you need to confront another member of your healthcare team. Identify the specific aspect of behaviour that needs to be modified in the other person. Plan your intervention, making sure that it is well timed and respectful of the other person, sandwiched with support on either side. Carry out your intervention and evaluate in terms of strengths and weaknesses. Do you need to repeat your confrontation in a different way?

4. Identify communication problems within your nursing or multi-disciplinary team. See if you can identify strategies for solving them, utilizing Heron's Six Category Intervention analysis. Remember that this model respects the autonomy of the other person, that is it recognizes the possibility that the other person may refuse to comply with the communication request and so the intervention may need to be repeated.

Degenerate Interventions from Heron's Six Category Intervention Analysis (1989)

The term 'degenerate intervention' has been used by Heron (1989) to describe those kinds of communication problems you have identified within your nursing or multidisciplinary team. If the patient is to be empowered through effective teamwork, communication problems within the team need to be ironed out. This relates to the idea of unconscious defence mechanisms operating in a collective manner to protect the team through institutionalised practices as identified by Menzies-Lyth (1988). Heron (1989) provides a useful framework for identifying communication problems within a healthcare team. If the model of six category intervention analysis is used correctly, it can resolve the three types of degenerate interventions listed below which can occur within teams:

1. *Unsolicited interventions*: these occur when someone intervenes before establishing that the other person wishes to be involved in an interaction.

2. *Manipulative interventions*: these occur when someone intervenes in order to satisfy their own interests rather than the interests of the other person.

3. *Compulsive interventions*: these are similar to the above but mean someone projects his or her own psychological material onto the other person and so loses sight of the true needs of the other person. Compulsive interventions are unconscious which means that the person lacks insight into their own behaviour and so are potentially more destructive.

Activities

1. Review the communication problems which you identified within your nursing or multi-disciplinary team for the last activity. Now categorise each communication problem according to the type of degenerate intervention.

2. Compare Heron's (1989) definitions of unsolicited, manipulative and compulsive interventions with Menzies-Lyth's (1988) unconscious defence mechanisms of splitting the nurse–patient relationship, depersonalization, detachment and denial of feelings, elimination of decisions by ritual task performance and collusive social redistribution of responsibility and irresponsibility.

3. Evaluate how much degenerate interventions and unconscious defence mechanisms within the healthcare team detract from your personal job satisfaction. Could you use Heron's (1989) Six Category Intervention analysis to improve communication within the team?

The Roles of Reflective Practice within Teamwork

Johns and Freshwater (1998) have written extensively on the role of reflective practice in enabling a nurse to improve the actual delivery of nursing care. Reflective practice emphasizes an experiential approach that is compatible with that of Heron's (1989). Six Category Intervention analysis as a model of communication strategies, which can enhance teamwork. The concept of the individual nurse reflecting on self within the practice context with a colleague or external professional in clinical supervision, links closely with the concept of the individual nurse analysing the communication context within the team so as to use the appropriate strategy. Reflective practice arises from humanistic psychology, which emphasizes the individual as conscious and able to exert personal agency or choice. It challenges the idea that unconscious communication needs determine nursing practice in teams as suggested by Menzies-Lyth (1988). Reflective practice gives individual nurses the tools to resist institutional practices, which function to protect healthcare teams from anxiety rather than to empower patients. As the individual nurse confronts the contradictions within his or her practice, the nurse becomes empowered to question and debate practices within the nursing and the multi-disciplinary teams in a constructive manner.

In a climate of clinical governance, Johns and Freshwater (1998) provide a reflective system for monitoring quality with reference to standards of care and a reflective review through clinical supervision. The dynamic interaction of healthcare professionals with very different roles results in multiple stories or narratives concerning both the patients and the healthcare professionals themselves. Reflective practice gives the individual nurse the opportunity to unravel some of these multiple stories, though how she or he makes sense of them will be influenced by the social context and, specifically, the relationship with a particular clinical supervisor. Reflective practice highlights the complexity of teamwork, as there may be conflict between the conscious, task-orientated agenda and the unconscious, emotional needs of the team. A reflective system can improve relationships within the nursing team by providing a positive culture for managing complaints and mistakes and a space for reflective debriefing.

There are advantages and disadvantages for the nursing team if clinical supervision is conducted by a line manager. The advantages relate to the potential for mutual growth and empowerment as nurses at different levels can work together to achieve shared goals. The disadvantages relate to power issues, with the potential for the manager to manipulate the individual nurse's agenda to fit their own purposes and the nurse may avoid discussing certain experiences, which are traumatic.

Conclusion

In a climate of clinical governance, team members need to identify their specific roles in order to work efficiently and effectively. Together with reflective practice, the nurse is enabled to unravel the multiple narratives in the dynamic interaction of healthcare professionals. This should enable the nurse to resist institutional practices that detract from the empowerment of patients.

7

Managing Diabetes

JOAN BENDALL and TESSA MUNCEY

Glucose can severely damage your health. (Hales, 1994)

This chapter outlines the impact of diabetes on the individual and describes the knowledge that is required to monitor the individual effectively. This includes protocols for clinics and auditing processes.

Diagnosis of Diabetes Mellitus

Diabetes is a metabolic disorder resulting from an absolute or relative lack of insulin, resulting in an inability to control the use and storage of glucose and, therefore, blood glucose levels rise. It is clinically characterised by the classic symptoms of thirst, polyuria, weight loss and biochemically characterised by a high blood sugar and, in some cases, ketosis. The system responsible for this imbalance is the endocrine system (see Box 7.1).

Box 7.1   **Criteria for the diagnosis of diabetes**

- Symptoms (which may include unexplained weight loss, thirst, polyuria, recurrent infections) are present with a random capillary whole blood glucose concentration greater than 11.1 mmol/l
- Fasting plasma glucose concentration $>= 7$ mmol/l on a minimum of two occasions where fasting is defined as no calorie intake for at least eight hours
- A two-hour plasma glucose concentration $>= 11.1$ mmol/l during an oral glucose tolerance test (OGTT) (The American Diabetic Association guidelines state that OGTT is not recommended for routine clinical use.)

Source: Alberti and Zimmet, 1998

The Endocrine System

The endocrine system is part of the chemical communication system of the body. It consists of a number of ductless glands, scattered throughout the body, that synthesise and store their chemical messengers, or hormones, and releases them directly into the blood in response to a stimulus. The hormones circulate around the body and interact with target organs, by binding to specific receptors and bringing about a response. Endocrine glands are stimulated to release their hormones either by other hormones (termed tropic hormones), humoral stimuli such as blood sugar or calcium levels, or neural stimuli. Negative feedback, that is the process that tends to cause levels of a variable to change in a direction opposite to the original change, is important in regulating hormone levels in the blood. Hormonally regulated processes include the stress response, maintenance of salt, water and nutrient balance, growth and development, and regulation of cellular metabolism. The main glands of the endocrine system are the pituitary, thyroid, parathyroid, pancreas, adrenals, ovaries and testes. Of particular concern to the management of diabetes is the function of the pancreas.

The Pancreas

The pancreas produces the hormones insulin, glucagon and somatostatin, as well as acting as an exocrine gland and releasing digestive enzymes into the duodenum. Insulin is produced by the pancreatic β-cells in response to increased blood levels of glucose, human growth hormone, adrenocorticotropic hormone and gastrointestinal hormones. Insulin is required for the entry, utilisation and storage of glucose, amino acids and fats by cells, and it exerts its effect by:

- stimulating the transport of glucose into cells
- stimulating glycogenesis (glycogen production) in the liver
- inhibiting glycogenolysis (glycogen breakdown) and gluconeogenesis (production of glucose from protein and fat)
- promoting the entry of amino acids into cells and stimulating protein synthesis
- stimulating lipogenesis (fat synthesis) and inhibiting lipolysis (fat breakdown).

The action of insulin is antagonised by glucagon, adrenaline, hydrocortisone, thyroxine and growth hormone.

Glucagon is produced by the α-cells of the pancreas in response to decreased blood glucose levels, exercise- and protein-rich meals. It serves to raise the blood sugar levels by accelerating glycogenolysis and gluco-neogenesis in the liver, and releasing glucose into the blood. The δ-cells of the pancreas secrete somatostatin or growth hormone inhibiting hormone (GHIH). This acts as a paracrine, or locally acting, hormone to inhibit the secretion of insulin and glucagon.

Pathophysiology of Diabetes Mellitus

Diabetes mellitus is an endocrine disorder, affecting 2 per cent of the population in the UK, in which the circulating levels of effective insulin are insufficient to maintain blood glucose concentrations within the normal range (that is 4–7 mmol/l) (Brown, 1998). The WHO (Alberti and Zimmet, 1998) recognizes five categories of diabetes, together with impaired glucose tolerance (see Table 7.1). However, of these categories, types 1 and 2 diabetes are by far the most common. The incidence of diabetes is increasing, especially type 2, and it is suggested that the world's diabetic population will have doubled from an estimated 110 million in 1994 to 221 million in 2010 (Orchard, 1998).

As can be seen from Box 7.2, type 1 and type 2 diabetes are two very different conditions. Type 1 diabetes is believed to result from an altered immune response to the insulin producing cells of the pancreas triggered by some environmental factor, for example a viral infection (Zimmet, 1993). Because of this response, the pancreas produces little or no insulin and so life-long insulin replacement is required. In type 2 diabetes, insulin is produced by the pancreas, sometimes at elevated levels. However, the body cells do not respond fully to the insulin, and oral hypoglycaemic agents or insulin may have to be given to improve the response and correct the hyperglycaemia. Type 2 diabetes has a strong genetic component and can be precipitated by obesity (Bingley and Gale, 1993).

If effective insulin is not available to the body cells, then two problems can develop (see Figure 7.1) First, glucose cannot be utilized for energy. Consequently the body cells have to use other energy sources and so they catabolise muscle and fat stores. This results in loss of weight, weakness and lethargy. The increased movement of fats around the body leads to hyper-lipidaemia and increased risk of atherosclerosis, with its complications of angina, coronary thrombosis, cerebral vascular accidents, peripheral vascular disease and gangrene. Mammalian cells are unable to totally metabolise fats to carbon dioxide and water without the presence of glucose. Instead, the end product of fat metabolism is ketones, which in

Table 7.1   WHO classification of diabetes

---

1. Insulin-dependent diabetes mellitus (IDDM) or juvenile onset diabetes – now termed type 1 diabetes

2. Non-insulin dependent diabetes mellitus (NIDDM) or late onset diabetes – now termed type 2 diabetes
   non-obese
   obese

3. Malnutrition related diabetes mellitus (MRDM) – also called tropical diabetes

4. Diabetes associated with other conditions and syndromes:
   pancreatic disease, e.g. pancreatitis
   diseases of hormonal aetiology, e.g. Cushing's disease
   drug, e.g. ritonavir, pentamidine or chemical induced diabetes, e.g. Vacor, a rodenticide
   abnormalities of insulin or its receptors
   certain genetic syndromes
   miscellaneous

5. Gestational diabetes – diabetes which occurs during pregnancy but reverts to normoglycaemia usually within six weeks of the birth

6. Impaired glucose tolerance (IGT) – fasting blood glucose above the normal range, but not within the diabetic range, i.e. above 5.7 mmol/l but below 11.1 mmol/l

---

Source: Alberti and Zimmet, 1998.

quantity are toxic and lead to ketoacidosis. Ketoacidosis is defined as plasma ketoacid levels greater than 10 mmol/l (Goguen and Josse, 1993) and is recognized by the smell of acetone on the breath, deep, rapid breathing (Kussmaul's respiration) and decreased consciousness (Higgins, 1994b).

Second, because the glucose, which is unable to enter the cells, remains in the blood it causes hyperglycaemia. The sugar is partially excreted in the urine where it exerts an osmotic effect leading to diuresis and dehydration. If not corrected with insulin, the dehydration combined with ketoacidosis and hyperglycaemia leads to coma and finally death. Even if the hyperglycaemia does not become severe enough to produce a coma, in the long term raised blood sugar levels cause glycosolation of tissues and precipitates many of the long term complications of diabetes, in particular microvascular and macrovascular disease, and cataract formation. Hyperglycaemia also inhibits the activity of the immune system and so predisposes to infections, the most frequently encountered being genitourinary and wound infections.

Table 7.2   Comparisons between type 1 and type 2 diabetes

	Type 1	*Type 2*
Age of onset	<20	40+
Type on onset	Abrupt, often severe	Gradual, usually subtle
Usual body weight	Lean and wasted to normal	Obese (80%)
Genetic risk	Weak	Strong
Beta cells	Markedly reduced	Normal or slightly reduced
Islet antibodies	Present	Absent
Islet lesions	Inflammation, atrophy, fibrosis	Fibrosis, amyloid
Blood insulin	Markedly reduced	Elevated or normal
Hyperglycaemia	Present	Present
Ketones	Present	Absent
Insulin sensitivity of cells	Sensitive	Relatively resistant

Figure 7.1   The physiology of the under secretion of insulin

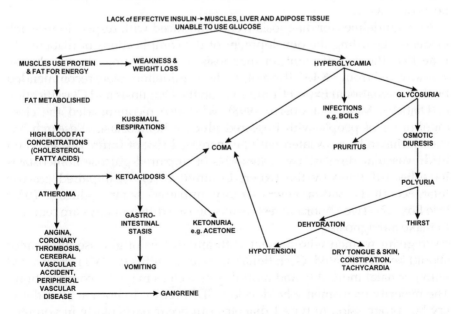

Source: reprinted from S. J., Hopkins *Drugs and Pharmacology for Nurses* (1999) 13th edn, p. 196 by permission of the publisher Churchill Livingstone.

Box 7.2 **Criteria for impaired fasting glucose and impaired glucose tolerance**

- IFG: fasting plasma glucose $\geqslant$ 6.1 mmol/l but < 7.0 mmol/l
- IGT: 2 hour plasma glucose during an OGTT $\geqslant$ 7.8 mmol/l but < 11.1 mmol/l

---

Diagnosis

The diagnosis of diabetes is based on the patient's clinical symptoms in combination with a measure of blood glucose levels (Higgins, 1994). As a diagnosis of diabetes has important legal and medical implications for the patient, it is vital that the diagnosis is accurate. Consequently, a diagnosis should never be made based on glycosuria or a stick reading of a finger prick test. The diagnosis must be confirmed by a glucose measurement performed in an accredited laboratory on a venous plasma sample with values of >11 mmol/l with symptoms and 12 without symptoms (MacKinnon, 1998 p. 61). Box 7.2 indicates the criteria for a positive diagnosis of diabetes.

New guidelines for diagnosis were announced with respect to research evidence regarding the development of the complications of diabetes. In June 1997 the cut off point for diagnosis using a fasting plasma glucose was lowered from 7.8 to 7.0 mmol/l. These guidelines were recommended by the International Expert Committee on the Diagnosis and Classification of Diabetes Mellitus (Alberti, 1998), who also recommended the close monitoring of people with impaired glucose homeostasis. Research has shown this to be associated with an increased risk of future diabetes and cardiovascular disease. Two categories of impaired glucose homeostasis have been defined by the Expert Committee (1997): impaired glucose tolerance (IGT) and a new category impaired fasting glucose (IFG) (see Box 7.2). Two abnormal test results on two different days are required to make a diagnosis.

Pregnant women who present with any degree of glucose intolerance should be investigated. Gestational diabetes mellitus (GDM) is associated with perinatal morbidity and mortality as well as maternal complications. The majority of women who develop GDM return to normal after delivery but progression to type 1 diabetes can occur particularly in younger, thinner patients. Alternatively, other women have an increased risk of developing type 2 diabetes in later life. It is recommended that women who develop GDM should be retested six weeks after delivery and reclassified according to the following four categories:

- Diabetes
- IFG
- IGT
- Normoglycaemia

The St Vincent Declaration

Recommendations for the management of diabetes mellitus were reached by representatives of Government Health Departments and patients' organisations from all European countries under the auspices of the WHO and the International Diabetes Federation in St Vincent, Italy on the 10–12 October (WHO, 1989).

Management Programme for Diabetes Mellitus

Earlier management of patients with diabetes required compliance with a strict regime of diet and drugs in a very restricted lifestyle. The paternalistic healthcare system ordered a strict regime of diet, drugs and healthcare monitoring. However, the eradication of long-term side effects was not possible because of the lack of understanding of the meaning of the disease for the patient and, therefore, their inability to adapt their lifestyle to the rigorous demands of the healthcare professional. If people are to fully understand the implications of the disease and are to be helped to manage it successfully then they must become partners in the diabetic management team. The team must acknowledge the potential hidden agendas for the person. (see Table 7.3).

Ken – a Case Study

Ken was a recently diagnosed insulin dependent diabetic. He was a business executive who commuted to work each day. At a recent company medical, he was found to be diabetic. The other feature of this medical was that he was overweight.

At his first follow up interview he said:

the dietician says my diet is fine, but I should lose weight and increase my exercise ...

Table 7.3   New diet advice for people with diabetes

- Avoid being overweight.
- The main part of each meal should be made up of high fibre, high carbohydrate foods.
- Eat less fat and exchange fats for polyunsaturated and non-saturated fats.
- Increase intake of fruit and vegetables to 400 g per day including 30 g of pulses, nuts and seeds (at least 5 portions of fruit and vegetables).
- A small amount of sugar (25 g) can be incorporated into a daily diet, low in fat and high in fibre.
- Special diabetic products are not necessary.
- Limit total salt intake to 6 g (around a teaspoon) a day – this includes salt contained in manufactured foods.
- High protein intakes should be avoided.

Obviously, this advice in the light of his diabetes and obesity is a contradiction, so careful listening reveals a hidden agenda. In talking about his diet he explained:

> After dinner each evening I like to share a bottle of port with my wife while we share the days activities before going to bed.

He had not included the port as part of his diet in discussion with the dietician. In light of this information, he was taught Blood Glucose monitoring. It was suggested he test his fasting blood sugar and two hours post meals for three days and one day pre meals. As he was starting in the 16–20 range, his first target was 10 fasting; the second target was 8 fasting aiming for a level of 5.5 to 6.5 fasting. As a result of his involvement in the monitoring, he experimented with his port intake, first by drinking a dry port and then changing to brandy that had less effect on his blood sugar. A gradual reduction in his drinking occurred as he made the positive move to lose weight.

Ken's story highlights that the objectives for the patient should be to empower them to live with diabetes by

- living confidently and participating in all normal activities while living with a progressive disease
- understanding some of the hurts and non-acceptance of diagnosis, which may have lasted in some instances for many years
- becoming valuable team members, enabling them to live long and healthy lives.

The team's objectives for themselves should be to have the confidence to interact with people who:

- appear to have all the answers
- who have lived with diabetes mellitus for most of their life
- where all professional advice has been ignored.

At whatever stage the nurse meets the person with diabetes for the first time, whether it is immediately following diagnosis or many years into management, the most important first step is to listen to their story.

Reaction to Diagnosis

Anybody who has recently been informed of the diagnosis of a chronic condition will be very distressed. Different coping mechanisms may come into operation. Initial reactions may vary between one of relief that there is a rational explanation for the variety of symptoms that they have been experiencing, to a feeling that it cannot be true. Relief may lead quickly to a desire to get involved, to get on with it, to find out what is involved but disbelief may manifest itself in a questioning of the diagnosis. Bewilderment may lead to panic and a difficulty in taking in more than immediate information. While initially the mind is very sharp taking in answers to questions such as 'what does it mean, what have I to do?' Almost simultaneously the mind is saying 'why me? It can't be true, this happens to other people not to me, I can't believe it.'

Initial reaction is masked then by the mind not wanting to accept the diagnosis and as one slowly realises that the condition will not disappear the denial is past and the shock sets in, quickly followed by fear of the unknown. Questions such as 'will I survive? What will it mean for my family, my children, for work? Can I drive my car? What have I done to deserve this? It's not fair? Why me? Following a period of introspection the person may take time to grieve for the self that might have been, as well as perceived changes in relationships with children, parents and grandparents. A feeling that life may never be the same, that they will never be the same, may lead to a feeling of being a second class citizen. Questions about the duration of the illness may lead to doubts about their ability to cope with it and confusion about what their priorities are. Consideration of lifestyle, family commitments, home, work and pleasure activities are important. If any crisis occurs in any of these area as, good diabetic control cannot be achieved.

Other influences on their reaction will depend on their own personal experience of the disease and people they have known or heard about with it:

> Tom who went into a coma and died from it when he was only 22 years old. Auntie Lizzy at Cleethorpes who went blind. Uncle George who had gangrene and lost both his legs, who had to inject himself every morning.

The bad experiences of injections as a child and the near certainty that it will be impossible to administer themself every day. However, despite all this distress, comforting words that reassure are not exactly what they want to hear, nor is it possible. People take different lengths of time to adjust to the point where they 'accept' the condition. Some may never be able to make this adjustment. Anyone who is distressed and trying to deal with difficult emotions will not be in the most receptive state of mind for 'education'. This needs to be kept in mind by the teacher and the information should be tailored appropriately. It is especially important in these early stages to actively listen to what is being said. Often there is a need to talk about feelings and have these acknowledged before information can be absorbed. It is important to remember the conditions, which enhance learning (see Box 7.3).

In the correct environment, a newly diagnosed person can be helped to incorporate the aims of good management into their lives (Box 7.4). The reasons for failure of these aims are failure to accept the truth of the diagnosis or lack motivation to review their lifestyle and incorporate new skills into their lives. Monitoring of the condition can be a pain both actually, as a result of blood glucose testing, and metaphorically in respect of disruption to an established pattern of living. One of the most important aspects

---

Box 7.3 **People learn better under the following conditions**

1. When they are listened to and responded to appropriately.
2. When misconceptions or outdated information has first been corrected.
3. When the information is relevant to them and their diabetes.
4. When they know the reasons why they are learning a particular thing.
5. When the information is built on existing knowledge.
6. When the information is clear and simple and ideally no more than two messages are given in any one session.
7. When the periods of teaching are not too long – ideally no longer than 10 minutes.
8. When the learning environment is relaxed and uninterrupted.

Box 7.4 **Aims of management of the newly diagnosed person with diabetes**

1. Come to terms with the diagnosis.
2. Include diabetes mellitus into their lifestyle.
3. Reduce anxiety.
4. Accept it will not go away.
5. Apply the information given.

to consider is the difficulty in accepting that complications will ever happen. Most people can cope with incubation periods of a few days between contact with an infectious disease and its onset with illnesses such as a cold or chickenpox. The idea, however, of many years intervening between the new diagnosis and the effects of complications, is difficult to grasp. Failure can be minimised by continuing reassure and reinforce to the message through answering the most persistent questions.

In the period immediately following diagnosis, it is important that a full medical examination and a range of information is given to the person. Given the wide range of information that is required to be absorbed it is useful if a close friend or relative can be involved in the informational sessions. An outline of the expectations for the person with insulin dependent diabetes is outlined in Box 7.5. The requirements of the person with non-insulin dependent diabetes are the same except for information about injection equipment. Instead, they will require instruction on blood or urine testing, what the results mean and supplies of relevant equipment.

Diet

One of the most important, conflicting and contentious pieces of information that a patient receives relates to food. Advice about diet is always changing; each person needs a personal food plan (see Table 7.3). Box 7.6 demonstrates the range of questions that people with diabetes need to become familiar with. Dietary advice may be given by a dietician who will need to establish what the person is used to eating and how it needs to be adapted. The person should be reassured that they can continue with many of their favourite foods, although incorporation of basic healthy eating measures will ensure better control and less long term complications.

Box 7.5 **Expectations of the person with newly diagnosed diabetes**

When they have just been diagnosed, they should have:

1. a full medical examination

2. an explanation of what diabetes is and what treatment they are likely to need: diet alone, diet and tablets, or diet and insulin

3. a talk with a dietician

4. instruction on injection technique, looking after equipment, blood glucose monitoring, ketone testing, supplies of relevant equipment and discussion about hypoglycaemia

5. a discussion about the implications of diabetes for their job, driving, insurance, prescription charges, and the need to inform the Drivers and Vehicle Licence Company and their Insurance company

6. information about Diabetes UK and any local groups

7. ongoing education about diabetes and the beneficial effects of exercise and regular monitoring of control

---

Hypoglycaemia

One of the greatest fears for the person with diabetes is a fall in blood sugar that may lead to a loss of consciousness. The resulting loss of self control that comes from not knowing when it may happen, the possibility of making a fool of themselves in front of friends or work colleagues makes this potential problem all the more worrying. They may have to face relatives and friends being embarrassed because they do not know what to do. The risk of hypoglycaemia at work may lead to disruption, accident risk and fear from those ignorant about the disease. Hypoglycaemia may have a very sudden onset and the symptoms themselves can be very frightening (see Box 7.7). The rate of the fall in blood sugar is one of the most important features to recognize because sudden loss of blood glucose can be the most difficult to deal with. The causes of hypoglycaemia may be taking too much insulin or oral hypoglycaemic medication, associated with poor timing of meals, too much exercise or a loss of body weight.

The treatment is to restore the blood glucose as quickly as possible by administering glucose, resting for 10 to 15 minutes and eating high fibre and protein food. During this time the blood glucose should be monitored regularly and if it falls below 4 mmol/l they should be encouraged to seek advice. Glucagon is a very effective treatment. It does not need to be given

---

Box 7.6　**Diet and diabetes quiz**

Are the following statements true or false?

	True	False
1 The carbohydrate content of foods is a good indicator of the blood glucose response to food	☐	☐
2 Increasing dietary fibre can have a blood glucose lowering effect in people with diabetes	☐	☐
3 Sprinkling bran on cereal is a good way of increasing dietary fibre intake	☐	☐
4 Digestive biscuits are a good snack to recommend	☐	☐
5 The recommendation for sugar consumption in people with diabetes is the same as for the general population	☐	☐
6 Special diabetic foods are recommended for people with diabetes	☐	☐
7 Sucron and sweet 'n' low are suitable sweeteners for people with diabetes to use	☐	☐
8 An important dietary recommendation for people with diabetes is the reduction in saturated fat intake from 17% energy (usual UK diet) to less than 10% energy	☐	☐
9 Cholesterol is the most important dietary factor in influencing blood lipid levels	☐	☐
10 A good intake of fruit and vegetables is important for a good intake of antioxidant vitamins	☐	☐
11 Approximately 75% of people with Type 2 are overweight	☐	☐
12 The dietary advice for Type 1 and Type 2 is in principle the same	☐	☐
13 There is a risk of hypoglycaemia occurring several hours after alcohol	☐	☐

Answers are given in Table 7.4

by a doctor. A supply of it can easily be kept at home and at work in the event of an emergency. Given sub-cutaneously or intra-muscularly it is equally effective and would be an ideal procedure to teach to a friend or relative. The adult dose of 1mg will raise circulating blood glucose by approximately 2mmol/l and will usually work within 10 to 20 minutes. However, glucagon is much less effective in alcohol-induced hypoglycaemia.

Table 7.4 Answers to diet and diabetes quiz (see Box 7.6)

		True	False
1	The carbohydrate content of foods is a good indicator of the blood glucose response to food	✓	
2	Increasing dietary fibre can have a blood glucose lowering effect in people with diabetes	✓	
3	Sprinkling bran on cereal is a good way of increasing dietary fibre intake		✓ It's OK but better to have a wholemeal cereal such as porridge or Weetabix
4	Digestive biscuits are a good snack to recommend		✓ High in fat, better to use an alternative such as fruit or sandwich with a low fat filling such as lean ham.
5	The recommendation for sugar consumption in people with diabetes is the same as for the general population	✓	
6	Special diabetic foods are recommended for people with diabetes		✓ They are expensive and contain Sorbitol which causes diarrhoea
7	Sucron and Sweet 'n' low are suitable sweeteners for people with diabetes to use		✓ These also contain Sorbitol as above. Better to Canderel or Sweetex
8	An important dietary recommendation for people with diabetes is the reduction in saturated fat intake from 17% energy (usual UK diet) to less than 10% energy	✓	
9	Cholesterol is the most important dietary factor in influencing blood lipid levels		✓ All fats influence blood lipid levels
10	A good intake of fruit and vegetables is important for a good intake of antioxidant vitamins	✓	
11	Approximately 75% of people with NIDDM are overweight	✓	
12	The dietary advice for IDDMS and NIDDMS is in principle the same	✓	
13	There is a risk of hypoglycaemia occurring several hours after alcohol	✓	

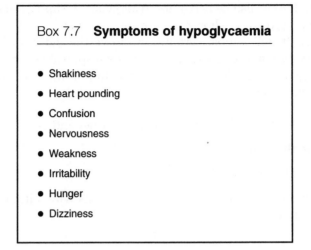

Box 7.7 **Symptoms of hypoglycaemia**

- Shakiness
- Heart pounding
- Confusion
- Nervousness
- Weakness
- Irritability
- Hunger
- Dizziness

Monitoring and control

Jo – a Case Study

Jo was a very bitter, angry young man in his late thirties, who had been a type 1 diabetic for 20 years. He denies that he is a diabetic and has only injected in his thighs for 20 years. He has only taken occasional blood sugars before bed and breakfast time when his out-patient appointment is due. He has a fear of sudden hypos and feels they ruin his life by a loss of self control and embarrassment. His main aim is to eat when and what he likes but he has a fear of having to inject up to four times a day. Resistance to any formal education stemmed from his fear that DM would rule his life. However, ironically because of his desire not to be controlled by the disease, he was in fact at the mercy of a very uncontrolled blood sugar.

Careful negotiation was required to encourage self help. Two ways were suggested: (a) investigate the appropriateness of his insulin mixture in the morning; and (b) stop monitoring before breakfast and bedtime but test at individual meal times whenever possible. Agreement with this minor modification to the regime was achieved, probably because he did not feel pressurised into expectations he could not keep. No dramatic improvements occur this way but gradual adjustments and increasing confidence result in lower glucose levels over time.

Jo's experience highlights a range of issues for nurses that good monitoring can improve. It is very important to monitor blood glucose, especially in the early days following diagnosis, to assess the effectiveness of treatment. It may also be necessary to allow for the appropriate adjustment of treatment during short-term problems such as illness or during pregnancy. It will almost certainly improve the individual's confidence and motivation and encourage them to be responsible for their own well being by giving them important feedback. Important sickness rules for the person with diabetes include:

- continue with your diabetes treatment (diet and tablets or insulin)
- ensure that you drink plenty of liquid
- test urine or blood 24 hourly
- if a loss of appetite occurs, substitute meals with a liquid or light diet e.g. soup or ice cream.

Glycosylated Haemoglobin (HbA1c)

As new red cells are formed, some of the haemoglobin (Hb), which is contained within these cells, combines with glucose. This portion of the total Hb is called glycosylated haemoglobin (HbA1c). The amount of HbA1c formed depends on the overall amount of glucose in the blood during the lifetime of the red blood cells, that is the greater the blood glucose, the greater the level of HbA1c. Therefore, because the lifespan of a red blood cell is approximately 120 days, the measurement of HbA1c at any given time will give some indication of the blood glucose level during the past 120 days.

Methods of Monitoring

Blood glucose testing is preferable for metabolic control. It is mandatory for patients on insulin and desirable for patients on oral anti-diabetic drugs, and is a vital safeguard against hypoglycaemia (Alberti, 1999). Monitoring can either be by testing blood glucose or urine testing. The advantages of blood glucose testing are:

1. virtually instantaneous measure of blood glucose level allowing immediate adjustment of treatment
2. instant diagnosis of hypo- or hyperglycaemia
3. fairly easy to perform with adequate training
4. unaffected by renal threshold to glucose

5. allows very tight control of blood glucose especially during illness or pregnancy.

Disadvantages of blood glucose testing are:

1. painful
2. requires good technique
3. more equipment needed
4. needs good eyesight
5. potential hazard from blood borne infection e.g. hepatitis.

Urine testing is an alternative method, which has the advantages of:

1. being simple
2. cheaper
3. needing less equipment.

However it has the disadvantages of:

1. not measuring blood glucose level
2. not detecting hypoglycaemia
3. some patients may find it distasteful
4. requires good eyesight
5. no meter available to overcome colour blindness
6. being affected by normal renal threshold. Note: the bladder should be emptied at least half-an-hour before a fresh specimen is collected and tested, otherwise the glucose level may be inaccurate.

Frequency of Monitoring

Frequency of monitoring will depend on whether the patient is well controlled and stable or poorly controlled and unstable. The frequency of testing blood glucose will depend on level of control – the better the control the fewer the tests. However, certain circumstances require more frequent monitoring. They include:

1. pregnancy
2. illness
3. unusual activity

4.   travelling

5.   multi-injection insulin therapy e.g. Novopen.

Urine testing is usually less frequent than blood glucose testing, but again frequency depends on individual control. Although optional for the person with type 2 diabetes there are advantages for blood monitoring. The individual can:

1.   take relevant action on knowing results

2.   aids compliance

3.   motivation

4.   learns how certain situations alter blood glucose levels

5.   warns them about hypo-hyperglycaemia

6.   less infections, improves healing, fewer skin problems

7.   security and confidence

8.   fewer days off work may lead to better career prospects

9.   nurses can use blood monitoring as an opportunity to improve overall knowledge of Type 2 diabetes for the patient

10. helps to prevent complications e.g. retinopathy, neuropathy, nephropathy

11. people with diabetes are responsible for their own health and well being.

When to Test

Blood Glucose

- before meals – reflects trough level before inevitable increase with food – more consistent

- after meals – measure of efficiency of insulin action.

Urine testing

- before meals – reflects overall glucose level during previous few hours while urine collecting in bladder

- after meals – reflects degree to which glucose level has risen following meal.

What Can Go Wrong with Monitoring?

The most common cause of error in blood or urine testing is poor technique. This can lead to inaccurate results being obtained. Poor technique includes not washing hands before testing, not using strips/stix correctly and not being trained properly to use the equipment they have been given or purchased. Most of these problems can be overcome by effective training. Other problems that may occur include using out-of-date strips or confusing the use of blood and urine sticks. Equipment may be faulty, for example, using the wrong strip for the meter if blood testing, or not having the meter calibrated or coded correctly. The user may not understand the reason for the test, which may lead to poor technique. Again most of these problems can be avoided with careful training and regular checks on technique and equipment. The recent introduction of more sophisticated equipment has helped to eliminate many of these problems.

Follow Up and Recall

After the initial diagnosis, a system of follow-up and recall needs to be negotiated. Ideally, appointments to monitor progress and identify early evidence of complications should, in the early stages, be every two to four weeks. As the condition stabilises this may be reduced to six monthly but the absolute minimum attendance to be encouraged should be for the annual review.

Separate records should be kept which ideally the patient should hold. This is essential for good care particularly where several team members are sharing that care. It can then be an easy reference for others and recall may be managed by a card index, a diary system or computer generated (see Figure 7.2).

Protocol of a Diabetic Clinic

The recall system should be part of an overall protocol for the management of people with diabetes in general practice (see Box 7.8). Clear guidelines must be agreed between the GP and the nurses involved, and appropriate training should be undertaken.

The protocol should:

1. set out the aims of the clinic

2. type of diabetes to be treated and appropriate treatment to be given, for example, perhaps only type 2 to be treated in the surgery, and the diet and oral therapy agreed

138

Figure 7.2 Flow chart to show a diabetic patient recall system

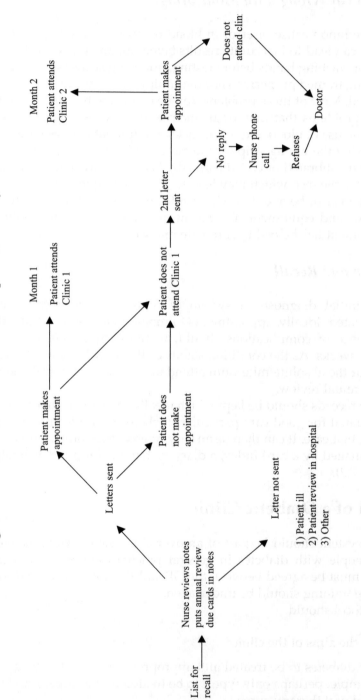

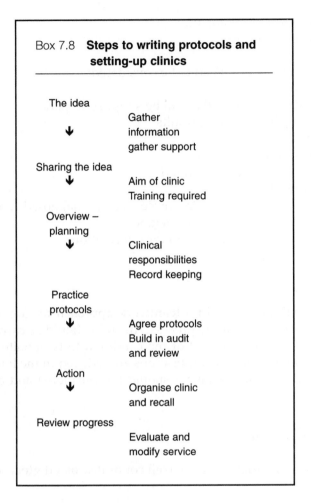

Box 7.8 **Steps to writing protocols and setting-up clinics**

The idea
↓   Gather information gather support

Sharing the idea
↓   Aim of clinic Training required

Overview – planning
↓   Clinical responsibilities Record keeping

Practice protocols
↓   Agree protocols Build in audit and review

Action
↓   Organise clinic and recall

Review progress
        Evaluate and modify service

3. an agreed timescale for alterations to treatment, for example, an over-weight type 2 patient may be given 3 months before considering oral therapy

4. establish frequency of visits to clinic 3-, 4-, and 6-monthly or annually.

5. approximate time for each consultation 15, 20 or 30 minutes.

6. screening and education to be carried out at each visit

7. when to refer for specialist treatment:
   a. proteinuria
   b. raised blood pressure

    c. background retinopathy
    d. hyperlipidaemia

8. The following also need to be considered:
    a. equipment
    b. leaflets and books that can be supplied to patients
    c. method of recording results
    d. recall system
    e. housebound patients
    f. patients who do not attend
    g. means of auditing
    h. standards of care, for example a newly diagnosed type 2 patient to be seen within 5 days of diagnosis
    i. Diabetes UK membership for information

Audit

One essential ingredient of a teamwork approach to care of the patient with diabetes is an auditing process. An audit should be carried out annually. This will enable control of the condition to be monitored regularly and determine whether complications are reduced in the long term. Each aspect of diabetic management should be considered and questioned in the following way:

Problem/Question 1

Do patients with diabetes have well controlled blood glucose levels?

Criteria

The fasting blood glucose levels of all patients should be in the range recommended in the district protocol for their age (e.g. 40–60 years: $< 8.5\,\text{mmol/l}$).

Re-evaluate

Confirm improvement next year.

Standard

90%.

Design and Implement Change

Highlight notes or recall patients with poor control. Improve dietary advice. Lower the threshold for starting tablets or insulin treatment.

Measure Performance and Compare Standard

Review the notes or make a random sample, check the level of blood glucose against this standard.

Problem/Question 2

Do patients with diabetes have an eye examination annually?

Criteria

As stated in the protocol all patients with diabetes should be offered an eye examination annually.

Re-evaluate

Confirm improvement next year.

Standard

90%.

Design and implement change

Individual patients who have not had an eye examination could be recalled or have their notes tagged for opportunistic screening.

Measure Performance and Compare Standard

Review the notes or a random sample, and check whether patients have had an eye examination in the past year.

Conclusion

The long-term patient with diabetes should become the 'expert patient'. They require a team approach to enable them to live a life devoid of long term complications with the flexibility to enjoy life to the full as independently as possible. The ritualised practice of a healthcare service that presumes to know what is best for the public and assumes compliance with its prescriptions must cease.

8

Living with Diabetes

JOAN BENDALL, JENNY KELLY and TESSA MUNCEY

The Diabetic patient must be his own Doctor, Dietician and Laboratory Technician thence education is the single most important aspect of treatment. (Lawrence, 1960)

To be given a diagnosis of diabetes is for most people a life sentence from which they cannot escape. This chapter will outline the team management of the patient with diabetes and consider the lifestyle issues that each individual must consider. The aim of treatment is to enable them to live confidently, participating in all normal activities while acknowledging that they have a progressive disease. Particular attention is paid to those lifestyle issues, whereby the person can be empowered to make their own decisions and so, become part of the team themselves.

In the early days of treating the person with diabetes, the nurse's role in caring for them was to administer the recommended drugs, ensure compliance with a strict dietary regime and carry out complex testing of urine. The complicated calculation of insulin with its different strengths of 40 and 80 and the glass syringes marked in 20 or 40 units ensured that the treatment remained for most a mystery. Dietary control was a complicated mathematical game of units and portions and diabetic ingredients with the occasional 'free' portion that the person could decide for themselves. Testing urine required chemistry laboratory equipment such as Bunsen burners, Feylings solution and Clinitest tabs. The focus of this treatment was not the individual patient and failed to recognize the needs, wishes and idiosyncrasies of them as distinctive human beings.

Recognizing the weaknesses in this approach to management of chronic diseases leads to a re-evaluation of the team approach. No individual's diet is the same every day; weekends may be different to weekdays, holidays will almost certainly be different to working life and there are not many people for whom Christmas and other religious festivals such as Ramadan does not mean during the former over indulgence and in the latter a desire to fast. It is this variety of difference that must be incorporated into a plan, which will work.

Initial Assessment

A very comprehensive initial assessment will pave the way to a successful long term relationship. Many of the investigations will serve as a base line for follow-up assessments. Follow-up will vary according to the needs of the individual, but should never be less than an annual review. Immediately following diagnosis may be a crisis time for the person and their family, and the information given should be clear and accurate. Arthur's story is an illustration of the need for careful explanations.

Arthur – a Case Study

Arthur was a very active gentleman, recently retired, whose diabetes was diagnosed at a routine visit to the surgery with blood glucose in the upper teens. The GP commenced him on an oral hypoglycaemic and finding a diet sheet in his drawer issued it to Arthur with minimal instruction.

Arthur's wife, keen to support him, insisted that they both follow it completely as she felt she needed to slim. After following the diet for two weeks, Arthur collapsed in town and following his third visit to A and E, a diabetes specialist nurse reassessed him. She took the time to listen to his story. His wife had responded to the diet sheet by eliminating carbohydrate completely. Therefore, he had been taking his oral hypoglycaemic with no carbohydrate balance. He had not been told to monitor his blood sugar and, therefore, the follow-up appointment for four weeks did not correct the problems.

Careful education about the role of complex carbohydrates, a diet avoiding added sugar, and teaching how and when to test his own blood glucose enabled Arthur eventually to discontinue his oral hypoglycaemic medication and maintain a normal range of blood glucose.

As well as personal history it is important to establish family history as this has implications for complications as well as the persons understanding of the treatment and monitoring approaches.

Mary – a Case Study

Mary was 60 years old and aware of her diagnosis of Type 2 diabetes as her mother had also had diabetes. She was taught how to test her urine using diastix, because her previous experience had been using clinitest, and was advised to reduce the sugar content in food only. She was requested to test for three days and then every third day, returning to clinic within one month. Tests changed from 2 per cent to 0.5 per cent glucose in that month. The change in blood sugar levels surprised her. When it was explained that the tests indicated that she was indeed reducing her sugar intake she became very angry.

> Why did no one tell me this when I was nursing my mother who lost her legs to gangrene and was never on a diet? I never knew that the colour of the urine test could change, it was always orange, and I just knew she had sugar.

Mary's story demonstrates the need to investigate the family history of a newly diagnosed diabetic in order to establish the level of prior knowledge and to identify areas that need updating or modifying in the light of new research.

Treatment

Following the diagnosis of diabetes, one of the first tasks is to establish the best course of treatment. The management of type 1 diabetes involves replacing the deficient insulin, balancing the dose against diet and exercise. Following the diagnosis of type 2 diabetes a person should have a three-month trial of dietary modification. If this is not successful, there then is a choice between the sulphonylureas and the biguanides.

Dosage of Insulin

As insulin is a polypeptide, it cannot be taken orally and requires subcutaneous injection. Insulin used to be extracted from the pancreas of cows and pigs. These animal insulin's differ slightly from human insulin in their arrangement of certain amino acids, but it is now possible to produce human-type insulin from enzyme-modified-pork insulin (H-emp), or by recombinant DNA technology from *Escherichia coli* (H-prb) and yeast cells (H-pyr). These human-type insulins are being used to an increasing extent, and although they are considered to have a potency comparable with that of standard insulins some care must be taken when transferring a patient from animal- to human-type insulin. Hypoglycaemia may occur during the changeover period without the patient experiencing the normal warning signs of giddiness, tremor and palpitation. Some authorities consider that these risks have been over exaggerated, although in some patients the problems with hypoglycaemia have been so great that they have transferred back to porcine insulin (Brown, 1998a).

Insulin can be given intravenously, intramuscularly and intraperitoneally, but the most practical and commonly used route is subcutaneously (McLellan, 1993). The rate of absorption of insulin can be increased by increasing the particle size (that is crystalline insulins are slower than amorphous) or by complexing the insulin with zinc or protamine (Neal, 1997). Insulin preparations are classified traditionally into short, intermediate and long acting. A recent innovation, insulin lispro has altered the shape of the soluble insulin molecule by changing around two of the amino acids to give smaller particles and so a more rapid acting insulin. It should be noted that all long acting preparations of insulin are suspensions rather than solutions and so should not be given intravenously, nor should insulin lispro be given by this route.

As well as the formulation, other factors can affect insulin absorption. Decreasing the volume of drug given increases the rate of absorption of insulin, while absorption is slower if the injection site is damaged by lipohypertrophy. Any factor, which alters the skin blood flow, either locally, for example massaging or warming the injection site, or generally, for example physical exercise, can hasten absorption. Minor differences also exist in the rates of absorption from different sites; it is fastest from the abdomen followed by the buttock, arm, thigh and calf (see Box 8.1).

It is important to choose the most appropriate insulin regimen for the patient (see Table 8.1). The younger the patient the higher the recommended number of daily injections, with the aim of strict, near normalisation of blood glucose (Slama, 1993). The client also needs to be taught to give the injection safely either using a needle and syringe or a multidose 'pen' injector. The skin does not need to be cleaned with an alcohol swab as this hardens the skin – using normal soap and water is sufficient. The skin should be pinched and the needle inserted at 90° to avoid the muscle (Jacques, 1993). The site of injection should be rotated to prevent lipohypertrophy. Insulin should be stored in the cool away from sunlight, which can present problems when on holiday in hot climates. Patients

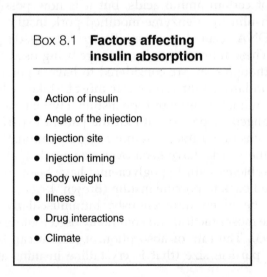

Box 8.1 **Factors affecting insulin absorption**

- Action of insulin
- Angle of the injection
- Injection site
- Injection timing
- Body weight
- Illness
- Drug interactions
- Climate

Table 8.1   Insulin injection regimens

Injection regimen	Comments
Once daily	Used for elderly patients where the District Nurse has to visit and give the injection
Twice daily	A mixture of short acting and intermediate acting insulins are given twice daily, e.g. 30% soluble with 70% isophane
Four times daily	Soluble insulin before each meal and a long acting insulin at night
Continuous subcutaneous infusion pumps	Only used for small number of highly motivated people

should also be warned that insulin interacts with other drugs. For example alcohol, β-blockers and monoamine oxidase inhibitors potentiate the effect of insulin, while corticosteroids, thyroxine and some diuretics such as frusemide antagonise it.

The total daily output of endogenous insulin from the islet cells is around 30–40 units. Many insulin deficient people need 30–50 units per day, some more some less. Usually two-thirds of the daily dose is given in the morning and one third in the evening. The starting dose is tailored to the individual; factors such as weight, occupation, exercise and blood glucose levels help to determine the dose. To prevent hypoglycaemia the initial dose of insulin should be small and gradually increased until the blood glucose level is satisfactory for the individual.

There are currently over 50 branded varieties of insulin on the UK market but they fall into four main categories, short (soluble), intermediate (isophane), fixed mixture and long acting (lente) (see Box 8.2). For a comprehensive guide to the onset, peak activity and duration of action of different insulin preparations, refer to monthly MIMS Index (Duncan, 2000).

Effect of Types of Insulin

Factors that affect insulin absorption besides the action of the insulin have implications for teaching the technique as well as information shared from the medical examination (see Table 8.2). Illness will increase the instability of the blood glucose, as the body requires different amounts of energy for healing. Drug interactions can be of two kinds. Alcohol, β-blockers and mono-aminooxidase inhibitors will potentiate insulin absorption. Antagonists include corticosteroids, diuretics and oral contraceptives.

Box 8.2 **Types of insulin**

Type of insulin	Fixed mixture	Soluble	Isophane
Onset	30 mins	30 mins	1 hour
Peak action	1–12 hours	1–3 hours	2–8 hours
Duration	14–24 hours	5–7 hours	18–20 hours
Comment	Many varied ratios of pre-mixed insulins available Less dose errors than 'free-mixing'	Only clear insulin can be used intravenously Often used with longer acting insulin i.e. isophane Free-mixing pre-mixed insulins basal bolus	Isophane insulin can be used alone once daily or twice daily Newly diagnosed or transferred from type 2 Often used with soluble insulin 'Free mixing' gives flexibility for younger patients Pre-mixed insulins form 10/90 to 50/50 for stable elderly patients Basal insulin – multiple injection regimen

Oral Hypoglycaemics

The alternative drugs to insulin, which are used to treat type 2 diabetes, are referred to as the oral hypoglycaemics. These include the sulphonylureas, for example tolbutamide and glibenclamide, which are the first choice of oral agents and account for 75 per cent of prescriptions. They exert their action by:

- increasing β-cell sensitivity to glucose and so increasing insulin release by the pancreas

- increasing the number of insulin receptors on the surface of body cells and so increasing glucose uptake

- stimulating lipogenesis with decreased plasma free fatty acids.

Table 8.2 Effects of types of insulin

Type of insulin	Soluble (short acting)	Isophane (intermediate acting)	Fixed mixture (short and intermediate acting)	Lente (long acting)
Example	Actrapid, velosulin	Isophane insulin, insulin zinc	Human mixtard 30/70	Human ultratard
Onset	30 mins	1 hour	30 mins	4 hours
Peak Action	1–3 hours	2–8 hours	1–12 hours	8–24 hours
Duration	5–7 hours	18–20 hours	14–24 hours	24–28 hours
Comment	Only clear insulin can be used intravenously Often used with longer acting insulin i.e. isophane 'Free-mixing' pre-mixed insulins basal bolus	Isophane insulin can be used alone once daily or twice daily newly diagnosed or transferred from type 2 diabetes management. Often used with soluble insulin 'Free-mixing' gives flexibility for younger patients Pre-mixed insulins form 10/90 to 50/50 for stable elderly patients Basal insulin – multiple injection regimen	Many varied ratios of pre-mixed insulins available Less dose errors than 'free mixing'	

Sulphonylureas may be expected to produce a lasting reduction in blood glucose of around 3 mmol/l, which is often sufficient to control the disease in many patients (Brown, 1998b). There is little difference in clinical efficacy between the different members of the group; the major difference is in pharmokinetics and duration of action. Some sulphonylureas, like chlorpropamide and glibenclamide are long-acting and so should be avoided if possible, especially by the elderly (Cantrill, 1997). Because the sulphonylureas have the ability to increase insulin release from the pancreas there is a real risk of hypoglycaemia, and the longer action hypoglycaemics are more likely to lead to this adverse effect. Chlorpropamide also has additional adverse effects not shared with the other sulphonylureas, namely hyponatraemia and an 'antabuse' reaction if the patient takes it with alcohol.

The sulphonylureas can interact with other drugs. Alcohol, chloramphenicol, clofibrate, mono-amino oxidase inhibitors, non-steroidal anti-inflammatory drugs, sulphonamides and warfarin can potentiate their hypoglycaemic effect, while some drugs, for example thiazide and loop diuretics and corticosteroids decrease the action of the sulphonylureas due to their ability to cause hyperglycaemia.

The biguanides are the second group of oral hypoglycaemics, metformin being the only example. They work by:

- slowing absorption of glucose from the gut

- enhancing insulin-mediated glucose uptake

- increasing insulin-receptor binding

- inhibiting gluconeogenesis and glycogenolysis

- causing weight loss, which makes them useful in obesity.

The major adverse effect of metformin is the risk of lactic acidosis. Clients have an increased risk of developing this adverse effect if they have renal impairment, because this allows the drug to accumulate. The other client group with increased risk are those who already have increased levels of lactate, that is patients with heart disease and poorly perfused tissues, and patients with liver failure who are likely to have reduced clearance of circulating lactate. Metformin can also cause taste disturbances, nausea and severe diarrhoea and vomiting, which can result in reduced compliance with therapy. In contrast to the sulphonylureas, metformin does not directly cause hypoglycaemia (McLellan, 1993a), as the client is running on his own pancreatic insulin, which can be suppressed if hypoglycaemia develops (Amiel, 1993). Table 8.3 gives a protocol for the management of type 2 diabetes.

Table 8.3 Protocol for treatment of type 2 diabetes

Non-obese → diet only → + sulphonylurea → +metformin → consider   change to insulin

Obese →diet only → = metformin → + sulphonylurea → consider change to insulin

---

Source: [RCN, 1992].

Prevention of Diabetic Complications

There is evidence that poorly controlled diabetes mellitus; both types 1 and 2 can adversely affect virtually every organ system in the body over a period of time. In the case of type 2 diabetes, the onset is so insidious that by the time it is diagnosed about 50 per cent of affected individuals have some evidence of tissue damage, raising the issue of whether diabetes mellitus should be more actively screened for (Turner, 1993). Table 8.4 identifies the signs and symptoms associated with long term diabetic complications.

There is increasing evidence that maintaining near-normal blood glucose levels and in particular sustaining a glycosylated haemoglobin level (HbA1c) of 7 per cent or less significantly reduces the risk of long term complications (Brown, 1998c). The Diabetes Control and Complications Trial (1993) studied 1441 patients with type 1 diabetes who were randomised either to continue their usual treatment or to adopt a more intensive insulin regimen that was designed to improve their blood sugar control. At the end of the follow up period (mean follow-up 6.5 years), the patients in the control and intervention groups had HbA1c levels of 9 per cent and 7 per cent respectively. The effect of this tightened glycaemic control was to reduce the risk of retinopathy developing by 76 per cent, to reduce the risk of neuropathy by 60 per cent, and to reduce the risk of nephropathy between 35 and 56 per cent. Similarly, the UK Prospective Diabetes Study Group (1998a) demonstrated that tight control of blood glucose concentration (target 6 mmol/l) in people with type 2 diabetes reduced the risk of microvascular disease, with sulphonylureas and insulin producing equally good results. However, there is the problem, particularly demonstrated in the Diabetes Control and Complications Trial (1993), that tight control means a higher incidence of hypoglycaemia, which can be both distressing and dangerous.

Hypoglycaemia is defined as a blood glucose concentration of less than 2.3 mmol/l, but symptoms sometimes occur before this level is reached (Higgins, 1995). It occurs most commonly during treatment with insulin, but can also be caused by sulphonylureas. Use of acarbose or metformin with a sulphonylurea may also induce hypoglycaemia, but treatment with

Table 8.4   Signs and symptoms associated with the common long term
diabetic complications

Complication	Signs and symptoms
Cardiovascular disease (Barnett, 1994)	Angina Hyperlipidaemia Hypertension Myocardial infarction Peripheral vascular disease, claudication and gangrene Stroke
Neuropathy – autonomic and somatic (motor and sensory) (Boulton, 1993; Funnell and McNitt, 1988; Macleod, 1993)	Absence of sweating (anhydrosis) leading to dry skin, callus formation, fissures on feet Altered blood flow regulation leading to 'warm foot' Small muscle wasting of feet Foot deformity, e.g. bunions, claw toes, Charcot changes Loss of sensation, often in stocking and glove pattern Pain Cardiovascular abnormalities including postural hypotension Gastrointestinal motor disturbances including dysphagia, delayed gastric emptying, nausea and vomiting, constipation, diarrhoea Difficulty with micturition and overflow incontinence Hypoglycaemic unawareness Impotence and retrograde ejaculation
Nephropathy (Carroll, 1994; Douglas *et al.*, 1998; Watkins 1993)	Proteinuria Albuminuria – micro (30–300 mg/24 hours) and macro (> 300 mg/24 hours) Hypertension End stage renal failure
Eye disease – retinopathy and formation (Eriksen and Kohner, 1993)	Background retinopathy – no deterioration in sight, but microaneurysms, haemorrhages Proliferative retinopathy – sight threatening Maculopathy Blindness Cataracts

diet, metformin, or acarbose alone does not (Appleton and Jerreat, 1995). The symptoms associated with hypoglycaemia are partially caused by adrenaline, released in response to falling blood glucose, which causes tremor, sweating and tachycardia. The effects of reduced glucose to the brain lead to behavioural changes including confusion, aggression and drunken gait, fitting, coma and death. In the light of this complication, and their reduced life span, there is some argument for tolerating a moderate degree of hyperglycaemia in the elderly.

Good glycaemic control is achieved by a combination of drug therapy, diet, and exercise. The diet recommended for people with diabetes is the same as that recommended to the rest of the population, that is:

- adequate energy to maintain a body mass index of 20–25
- 50% of energy to be provided by high complex carbohydrates
- 10–15% of total energy from protein
- fat to be restricted to 30–35% of total energy
- alcohol intake should be minimal, and avoided in overweight patients, those with hypertriglyceridaemia, and/or hypertension (Toeller, 1993).

As well as good glycaemic control, other actions can be taken to reduce long term diabetic complications which include full assessment at the annual review (Table 8.5).

Patients with diabetes are two or three times more likely to develop cardiovascular disease than the normal population (Gibbs, 1993). One of the factors, which contribute to accelerated development of atherosclerosis, is hyperlipidaemia. A UK survey found that 28 per cent of patients with diabetes had hyperlipidaemia, but that it was not entirely attributable to poor control of diabetes, as 71 per cent of the hyperlipidaemic patients had an HbA1c value of less than 10 per cent (Paterson *et al.*, 1991). Thus, good glycaemic control alone will not overcome the problem. Other independent factors leading to hyperlipidaemia are age, obesity and renal impairment in type 1 diabetes, and abdominal obesity (high waist/hip ratio) and insulin resistance (Gibbs, 1993). Hyperlipidaemia can be improved by weight loss, low fat diet, regular exercise and lipid lowering drugs.

One of the effects of hyperlipidaemia can be to precipitate hypertension, and in patients with type 2 diabetes this condition is common, with a prevalence of between 40 and 60 per cent over the age range of 45–75 (UKPDS, 1998b). It has been known for some time that the progression of established nephropathy is reduced, or might even be halted, by intensive treatment of hypertension (Watkins, 1993). However, the UK Prospective Diabetes Study Group (1998b) has now shown that patients with hypertension and type 2

Table 8.5 Minimising the complications of diabetes mellitus

Good glycaemic control

Reduce blood pressure to below 140/90 mmHg – ACE inhibitors are first choice in patients with microalbuminuria; β-blockers, calcium channel blockers and diuretics can also be used singly or in combination (Douglas *et al.*, 1998).

2-yearly ophthalmoscopy so lesions can be detected early and treated with photocoagulation

Regular exercise to lower insulin resistance

Weight reduction to attain normal weight for height, that is body mass index of 20–25

Diet – limit calories from fat to 30% of total energy intake; increase polyunsaturates and reduce saturates, aiming for a P/S ratio of 2; increase use of monounsaturated oil, for example olive oil which increases high density lipoproteins (HDLs)

Lipid-lowering drugs should be considered to improve lipid profile – resins, HMG CoA reductase inhibitors, fibrates

Foot care education – wash and inspect feet daily, keep skin moisturised, avoid going barefoot, wear good fitting shoes, cut toenails straight across and consult a chiropodist if there are foot problems

diabetes assigned to tight control of blood pressure (a mean over 9 years of 144/82 mmHg) achieved a significant reduction in risk of 24 per cent for any end points related to diabetes, 32 per cent for death related to diabetes, 44 per cent for stroke, and 37 per cent for microvascular disease. In addition, there was a 56 per cent reduction in risk of heart failure. The study also identified that a β-blocker (atenolol) and an angiotensin-converting enzyme inhibitor (captopril) were similarly effective in reducing blood pressure complications (UKPDS, 1998c). Thus, blood pressure reduction in itself may be more important than the drug used.

Annual Review

The annual review is important to ensure the continued well being of the patient and to monitor for the most common complications.

Patients expectations

The annual review is an opportunity to reassess the patient's progress. The discussion should include their blood glucose control, an opportunity to

```
┌─────────────────────────────────────────────────┐
│  Box 8.3   Observations at annual review         │
│                                                   │
│  Observations        Comments                     │
│  ─────────────────────────────────────            │
│  Urine               tested for ketones           │
│                        microalbinuria             │
│  Weight              should be recorded           │
│  Blood               HbA1c, creatinine,           │
│                        cholesterol                │
│  Blood pressure      checked                      │
│  Vision              visual acuity fundoscopy     │
│                        or retinal photos          │
│  Legs and feet       Circulation and              │
│                        nerve supply               │
│  Injection sites     examine if on insulin        │
└─────────────────────────────────────────────────┘
```

express their concerns and recent results of their home monitoring. The same procedure should be followed whether in a primary care setting or a hospital clinic, the patient will then feel confident with the procedure (see Box 8.3). A number of observations and measurements will be taken and recorded and any deterioration will be treated or referred to the appropriate team member.

Risk Factors

Particular patients may be more at risk than others may and particular attention should be given to patients who meet the following criteria: a family history of diabetic problems or a persistently high HbA1c and also patients who persistently ignore hospital appointments or keep away from the surgery.

A test of albinuria levels should be offered once a year to all patients with type 1 diabetes who are between 12 and 70 years old and to all patients with type 2 from the time of diagnosis. The relative risk of renal impairment due to raised albinuria is shown in Box 8.4.

An important feature of the annual review is not only to promote optimum health but also to help the patient become responsible for themselves. As Margaret's case demonstrates it is too easy to make the patient dependent on the professionals.

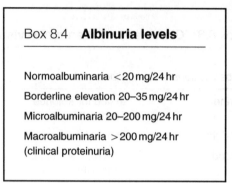

Box 8.4   **Albinuria levels**

Normoalbuminaria < 20 mg/24 hr

Borderline elevation 20–35 mg/24 hr

Microalbuminaria 20–200 mg/24 hr

Macroalbuminaria > 200 mg/24 hr
(clinical proteinuria)

Margaret – a Case Study

Margaret is a retired secretary and teacher and has lived with diabetes for 20 years. At a recent review four areas were identified that were worthy of further discussion.

1. Her lack of awareness of the meaning of poor control and the ability to influence the control by monitoring results.
2. Her awareness of complications and acceptance of her neuropathy and retinopathy as inevitable.
3. Her husband's awareness of when she feels unwell. From the discussion he did not mean hypoglycaemic attacks, as she had never had any, but the effect of hyperglycaemia on Margaret's temperament.
4. She deeply resents professionals telling her what to eat.

It would appear that after 20 years Margaret is very competent in everything but her diabetes. She is still reliant on professional expertise in telling her how and when to adjust her treatment despite demonstrating up to date knowledge about her condition. This would appear to be lack of confidence in applying the knowledge to herself despite being resentful of being told how to live her life. Time spent with Margaret increasing her confidence would give her back vital control over her life and minimise the inevitability of side effects.

Eye Care

Eye complications are frequent in diabetes and can lead to partial or even total loss of vision. However, much of this visual loss can be prevented by early detection and treatment. Cataract is twice as common in people with diabetes than in people without the condition, but can be effectively cured by surgery. The most severe complication, however, is diabetic retinopathy. This is a progressive disease involving the retina – the light-sensitive part at the back of the eye, which picks up the images, like the film in a camera. Adequate treatment by laser photocoagualtion can lower the risk of blindness but often diabetic retinopathy does not cause loss of vision until it is almost too late to intervene. In other words, patients with diabetes have sight-threatening retinopathy and are unaware of it. The only way to reduce the risk of loss of vision is to have the eyes checked regularly.

A two-yearly examination is usually sufficient to reduce the chances of loss of vision, as diabetic retinopathy has a relatively slow progression. However, in some cases, more frequent visits may be necessary particularly during pregnancy or prolonged illness. When recommending the patient to attend for an eye test it is important to encourage them to report any family tendency to high blood pressure, glaucoma or recent changes to vision and for the professional to explain the special nature of retinal screening and visual acuity. Examination to prevent diabetes-related blindness should include testing of visual acuity, dilatation of the pupils with eye drops and examination of the retina.

Visual Acuity

Visual acuity is a simple test. It indicates the acuteness of central vision for distance, near or reading position. In patients with diabetes mellitus normal visual acuity may be shown even though diabetic retinopathy is seen at fundoscopy. The test is important because normal to good vision is important in the self management of the condition. Good eyesight is needed for the following:

- checking of monitoring strip
- checking of insulin doses
- checking tablets taken
- inspecting feet
- checking skin lesions and injection sites
- reading specific instructions and educational material.

The check involves a fundoscopy examination with dilated pupils. In order that an accurate assessment is made a nurse will be required to ensure the following:

- adequate illumination
- ascertain that the patient is literate and speaks English

- spectacles or contact lenses must be worn if normally worn for distant vision
- each eye is tested separately
- use a clean plastic occluder for each patient
- allow time for the second eye to adapt to the light.

If the patient memorised the letters, change the chart or ask the patient to read the line backwards. If the patient cannot speak English or is illiterate their vision may be assessed using a Snellen E Chart. For young children who have not reached reading age a Kay picture test or Sheridan Gardiner chart is used.

Testing for Visual Acuity

The nurse can test visual acuity during the annual review using the procedure outlined in Box 8.5 and Box 8.6. If the patient cannot read the top letter of the chart at a distance of 1 metre then a visual check can be made using counted number of fingers. If the vision is considerably weaker than this an assessment of vision is made by holding the hand in front of the eye at 30 cm. If the patient cannot see hand movements, shine a bright pen torch intermittently into the eye, this may then be recorded as 'perception of light' or if there is no response 'no perception to light'. If the vision is

---

Box 8.5 Step by step procedure for testing visual acuity

1. Note whether glasses are worn.
2. Explain procedure to patient.
3. Place the patient facing the chart at the 6 metres (20 feet) or 3 metres (10 feet) mark.
4. Cover the left eye with an occluder (preferably plastic or plain card, never fingers or hand).
5. If the patient wears spectacles for distance vision keep them on.

Always test the right eye first

   (a) to facilitate recording
   (b) to avoid confusion.

Box 8.6 **An example of a recording**

(R)	VA	(L)
6/24	S	6/9
6/9	C	6/6
6/6	ph	6/6

---

found to have deteriorated a test using a pinhole occluder may be used to exclude errors or refraction.

The Pinhole Test

The pinhole test is used to differentiate between refractive and pathological visual loss and should be done routinely on all patients with a score of 6/9 or less. The same procedure is followed as above but an occluder is used with a small pinhole in its centre close to the tested eye. The visual acuity is recorded with a pinhole beside the reading. If the reduced visual acuity is related to a refractive error then the patient will usually be able to read considerably further down the chart with the pinhole. The pinhole works by only allowing the rays of light close to the principle axis through to the retina. These rays require very little refraction and are relatively unaffected by errors in the patient's optical system. If the visual acuity is improved using a pinhole, visual deterioration is due to poor focusing and an optician's assessment is required and corrective action taken. If the score is not improved then some other cause must be looked for.

Refractive Errors

It is important to remember that during stabilisation with medication – tablets or insulin – visual disturbances such as blurred vision may occur. This should be explained to the patient, as well as reassurance given, that the symptoms will settle, once blood glucose levels approach normality. During this period it is advisable not to visit the optician, waiting until their eyes have settled. This may take weeks or months but considerable inconvenience and expense may be incurred if the patient has not been informed of this problem.

The following abbreviations are used to record the visual score:

VA – visual acuity
C (cum) – with glasses

S (sine) – without glasses
ph – pinhole
CF – counting fingers
HM – hand in front of eye
PL – perception of light
NPL – no perception of light

If the visual acuity is found to have deteriorated during the annual review the patient should be advised to go to the opticians for a further check.

Other eye conditions associated with diabetes include cataracts, which may occur at a younger age in the patient with diabetes. Vitreous haemorrhage and retinal detachment may be a late consequence of proliferative diabetic retinopathy. Laser treatment may save the sight if retinopathy is present but requires urgent referral. Retinal vein occlusion is associated with diabetes, hypertension and a condition known as rubeosis of the iris may result in glaucoma. Rubeosis is the pink discoloration of the iris due to new blood vessels growing on the surface of the iris.

Foot Care

Attention must be paid to the feet because changes brought about by the diabetic condition make them vulnerable to several problems. Due to a combination of the blood vessels becoming narrower and a consequent lack of sensitivity, the foot becomes vulnerable to injury and subsequently to infection. In order to keep feet healthy it is quite important to wash the feet in warm water, dry them gently but thoroughly, rubbing in moisturising cream, and during this procedure inspect them for blemishes of damage. If the patients cannot do this themselves then they might ask a relative or friend to carry out the procedure.

Choosing comfortable footwear can protect feet, if the shoe is long enough, deep enough and wide enough. Shoes where the toes are squashed or that are too loose can cause damage. Well fitting shoes are preferable to slippers, and walking barefoot should be avoided. Socks too should be either cotton or wool and again should fit properly. It is possible for the patient to continue to cut their own toenails while they are easy to cut. They should be trimmed straight across and not to short. However, a chiropodist should be consulted if the patient has eyesight problems, loses feeling in the feet, or has poor circulation. A chiropodist should treat all corns and calluses and the patient should be discouraged from using medicated corn pads, lotions and ointments. People with diabetes are eligible for free treatment within the health service.

If small cuts and abrasions do occur they can be treated at home by cleaning the affected area and covering it with a clean dry dressing, which should be reapplied daily. Every day the wound should be checked to make sure it is healing and the chiropodist should be contacted if any of the following signs occur.

Danger Signs

- a small cut or abrasion fails to heal in a few days
- if there is extensive or deep injury
- colour change – if toes or feet change colour
- swelling
- discharge – infection my get into the wound
- pain – people with diabetes may have an altered sense of pain so if any of the above are present but are not particularly painful still encourage the patient to seek expert advice.

Employment

People with diabetes are encouraged to live a normal life, which for those under the age of retirement will mean work of some kind. Not everybody is well informed about diabetes and employers may be suspicious of employing somebody with diabetes because they are afraid they will be unreliable. Alternatively they may press them to become registered disabled to enable them to meet their quota. While it is commendable to encourage the person with diabetes to live a normal life their life is anything but normal following diagnosis. In addition to the physical requirements of the condition such as medication, injections and the need for constant monitoring, driving licences may be restricted and visits might need to be made to clinics or surgeries. The employee may need to adapt their diet and medication to changing shift patterns.

Diabetes UK (formerly The British Diabetic Association) has leaflets available aimed at employers to deal with concerns they may have. People with diabetes should always check the veracity of statements about diabetes made by employers advocating that they are affected by changes in policy or Health and Safety Regulations. Encourage the person to ask for an exact reference so that it can be checked. There are some jobs that are not open to those with diabetes. This may cause frustration and upset to someone who particularly has his or her heart set on a particular occupation.

Driving

It is a legal requirement to declare diabetes to the Drivers and Vehicle Licensing Centre (DVLC). The Road Traffic Act provides that any condition, which is expected to last for more than three months, must be declared. The exception being diet-controlled diabetes, which does not need to be declared. Changes of treatment must, however, be reported. In addition, the DVLC recommends that gestational diabetes, which is treated with insulin injections, should also be declared. Licences are generally restricted to three years where diabetes is treated by diet plus insulin. Where it is treated by diet alone, or by diet and tablets, an 'until 70' licence is used or maintained. Licences may be restricted to one, two or three years, depending on the medical report. The most common restriction is three years. Women with gestational diabetes who are treated with insulin do not have their licences restricted unless the condition persists six weeks after the birth of their baby.

There is no charge for licence renewal below the age of 70 years. After the age of 70 years, all drivers must pay a charge to renew their licence that can last for one, two or three years. All drivers should be advised of the need to inform the DVLC. It is an offence to drive with a prescribed disability without informing the DVLC and doing so can result in prosecution.

Refusal of a Licence

Apart from a 'hypo' at the wheel, reasons for revoking a licence include when a vocational licence holder reports treatment with insulin and when a driver or doctor reports loss of warning signs of hypoglycaemia or a deteriorating field of vision. The latter is often discovered when a test for field vision is requested after laser treatment has been reported on a DVLC medical form. Whatever the circumstances, the DVLC writes to the individual advising them not to drive, and to their GP advising of the reason for the revocation or refusal of a licence. Individuals should be advised to contact the GP in the first instance for further advice. GPs can inform the DVLC if the patient refuses to stop driving. There is a right of appeal to the Magistrates Court. Details of these are given in the letter of revocation or refusal.

Procedure for Renewing a Licence

The DVLC sends renewal papers to the individual 56 days before the licence expires. Once these forms are returned, the DVLC decides whether a further, medical report is required. If not, the licence is reissued based on their self report. At present, Vocational Driving licences cannot be renewed for those who are taking insulin. Driving is permitted while the licence is being renewed or while medical opinion is being sought.

The Procedure for First Time Applicants with Diabetes to Obtain a Driving Licence

Application for both a provisional and a full driving licence is made on the usual form, which asks about the presence of medical conditions. Where diabetes is noted, the DVLC sends the driver form 'Diabetic 1' to complete. This asks for details of the treatment and control of diabetes, as well as the name of the doctor(s) involved in the care. There is a consent form for the individual to sign, giving permission for DVLC to contact the doctor(s). Depending on the outcome of these reports, the licence may then be issued.

It is against the law for those on insulin to be issued with a Vocational Driving Licence that is a Large Goods Vehicle or Passenger Carrying Vehicle Licence, although this is currently under review. An expert panel is putting together an assessment model which will not discriminate against people who have well-controlled diabetes. The assessment will include the following criteria.

- There should be no disabling hypoglycaemia.
- They should have good awareness of hypoglycaemic symptoms.
- Their diabetes should be under regular (at least annual) specialist review.
- Their diabetes should be under stable control.

All insurance companies should also be advised of all forms of diabetes, including gestational and diet controlled diabetes. A policy can be rendered void if, when a claim is made it transpires that diabetes ('a material fact') has not been declared. The attitude of insurance companies varies, but loading is common, and is often made on the basis of insulin dose, and without any evidence of extra risk or problems. People are advised to shop around, challenge any excess loading either personally or through the Diabetes Care Department of Diabetes UK and, if necessary, to use their appointed brokers.

Travelling

Diabetes may add another dimension to apprehension to travelling abroad. However, as with any successful trip a little forward planning will alleviate most of the problems. Whatever one's state of health, it always makes sense to take out travel insurance which includes medical cover. Those intending to traveller should declare that they have diabetes, check the small print on the proposal form to make sure the condition is not specifically excluded, and look for minimum cover of £250 000. Diabetes UK is always pleased to give additional advice. In addition, if the destination is a country within the European Union an E11 form entitles the holder to emergency medical care. The form is available from the DSS offices as part of the Department of Health leaflet T1 'Health advice for travellers' and Post Offices; Leaflet T4 'The Travellers Guide to Health', is also useful.

There are no contraindications to vaccination or immunisation in people with diabetes, although they should be advised that control of their condition might be temporarily affected. Important items to be included in the packing when travelling include:

- diabetes identification
- insulin and syringes or oral hypoglycaemic agents
- needle clipper and disposable container
- other medication
- blood or urine monitoring equipment
- glucagon for those on insulin (glucagon hydrochloride is the hormone, which raises the blood sugar)
- fast acting carbohydrates.

Depending on the destination the following could also be appropriate:

- hypostop
- travel sickness prevention
- antidiarrhoeal medication
- anti-malarial medication
- simple dressings.

Not only is it advisable for extra supplies of insulin and equipment to be taken, but also, if travelling with somebody, split the supplies to avoid total loss. Always make sure that medications and equipment are carried in the hand luggage. This not only minimises the risk of loss, but also ensures that the drug is kept at the proper temperature. At high altitudes, insulin will be rendered inactive when the unpressurised holding cargo reaches freezing point while in flight. In addition, the blood strips will under read.

Meal Times and Food Quantities on the Journey

If a person with diabetes is familiar with what to eat they may be advised not to select the special diabetic diet from the menu but instead select from the normal menu. They may find themselves with insufficient carbohydrate in their special meal. However, it is always advisable to carry extra carbohydrates such as biscuits or fruit drinks to prevent possible hypoglycaemia. A further concern is juggling diet and medication while flying through different time zones. As a rule of thumb if the traveller loses time in a journey they may miss an injection or take less insulin on the day of arrival; if they gain time they may need an extra injection of short acting insulin.

At the holiday resort insulin may be stored in a refrigerator but it will remain stable at room temperature for up to one month in a dark place. In a warm climate everybody is advised to protect themselves from the sun, while the person with diabetes should particularly avoid burning and should use a high factor sun cream. Attention to footwear should continue as at home with well fitting shoes even on the beach to avoid injury particularly for those people with neuropathy.

In a warm climate insulin absorption may be faster, so hypoglycaemia is more likely. Regular checking in the first few days, with consequent reduction in insulin where necessary, should reduce the risk. It may be considered important that the person's travelling companion, where appropriate, should learn to administer glucagon as necessary, to avoid the necessity of emergency medical treatment. If the diabetic becomes ill on holiday particularly with diarrhoea and vomiting it is important that they continue with their treatment. Regular monitoring and alterations to treatment should be made until the condition subsides. If the blood sugar becomes higher than 17 mmol they should also check their urine for ketones. To avoid dehydration and hypoglycaemia it is advisable to drink fruit juices or sweetened drinks.

Team Involvement

During the course of their lifetime and while diagnosed as a diabetic, there will be interaction with a variety of healthcare professionals. The team responsible for the management of the person with the condition will not only be made up of members from primary and secondary care environments but most importantly people from home and possibly working environments (see Box 8.7).

Box 8.7 **Team members involved in the management of diabetes**

Home

Patient and spouse or main carer

Family, extended family, partner, friends

Care assistants in long stay hospitals/nursing homes/homeless night shelters/voluntary carers

Colleagues at work/occupational health nurses

Primary care

General Practitioner, practice nurse, receptionist, counsellor

Pharmacist, dietician, chiropodist optician, dentist

Social Services, Government agencies dealing with benefits, Drivers and Vehicle Licensing Centre, insurance companies, Diabetes UK

Secondary care

Dibetologist, consultant and the medical team, specialist nurses, specialist dietician

Clinic team – staff nurses, enrolled nurse, care assistants, receptionists

Other specialist team members – geriatrician, ophthalmologist, sister and staff in the eye clinic, eye ward

Foot care specialist, specialist chiropodist, and shoe fitters

Orthopaedic consultant, physiotherapists, occupational therapists

Renal unit

Dermatologist

Psychologist, psychiatrist

Pharmacy

Phlebotomist

Liaison staff between hospital and home

Patient Held Records

The wide variety of team members involved provides a real challenge to record keeping and continuity of care. Given that the patient should be a partner in the process of care and is always the link with all the other people, patient held records should be considered.

Conclusion

Diabetes is a complex disease that patients have to live with. Practice nurses have a vital role to play in helping these people to come to terms with their disease and to manage it effectively so that they can lead a relatively normal healthy life. In order to do this, the practice nurse must understand the disease and be aware of the latest research on its management, so that clients can be kept fully informed.

Part IV

Compliance in Chronic Disease Management

9

Compliance

JENNY KELLY

What is Compliance?

Non-compliance drastically lessens a patient's chances of attaining optimum health and because one of the main goals of nursing is to assist patients in attaining optimum health, the resolution of the problem of non-compliance is an important issue for nursing (Pfister-Minogue, 1993). But, what is compliance?

Compliance is classically defined as 'the extent to which a person's behaviour, in terms of taking medications, following diets, or executing lifestyle changes, coincides with medical health advice' (Haynes, 1979). Inherent in this definition is the belief that medical advice is 'good' for the patient, and that rational patient behaviour means following medical advice precisely. However, as the aim of compliance, particularly in chronic illness, is a well-controlled disease state, a more useful definition may be following medical advice sufficiently to achieve the 'therapeutic goal' (O'Hanrahan and O'Malley, 1981). This definition is closer to patients' ideas of compliance, as they define it in terms of apparent 'good health', and they seek treatment approaches that are manageable, liveable, and in there view effective (Roberson, 1992). However, this perspective may be flawed if it is based in the present, so that the long-term effects of the disease are not taken into consideration, and if it is based on limited knowledge due to the patient not being fully informed of all aspects of the condition and treatment.

Psychological Perspective

Psychologists have studied the issue of compliance or conformity for many years. They define compliance as a form of social influence in which an individual outwardly conforms, to obtain a reward or avoid punishment, but does not necessarily believe in the opinions expressed or the behaviours displayed. Studies show that situational factors can exert considerable influence over compliance (see Box 9.1).

Box 9.1 **Conformity**

Asch (1956) carried out an experiment in which a group of people seated around a table were shown a card with a vertical line on it together with a second card with three lines on it. In turn, the individuals were asked to identify which of the three lines was the same length as the single line. The judgements were easy to make and on most trials everyone gave the same answer. However, all except one of the group were accomplices of the experimenter, and on certain rounds they were all asked to give the same incorrect answer. To Asch's surprise, the subject of the experiment, who was always asked for his opinion last, gave the incorrect answer and conformed to group pressure approximately 32 per cent of the time, although he clearly knew he was giving the wrong answer, and 74 percentage of subjects conformed at least once. See Hilgard *et al.* (1979) for more details.

Box 9.2 **Utilizing cognitive dissonance theory to bring about behaviour change**

Janis and Mann (1965) asked women who were known smokers to play the role of a cancer patient. A doctor told each woman that he had some bad news. She had lung cancer and would have to undergo immediate surgery. The women played out the part by asking questions about the surgery, its likelihood of success, post-operative care, etc. The researchers followed up the women who had been involved in the role play and found that, compared to women who had listened to a tape recording of similar information, they had drastically reduced their smoking.
  See Coon (1983) for more details.

From the perspective of health education, compliance as defined by psychologists is insufficient, and what is required is internalisation. This occurs when a person believes the new opinions or behaviours and incorporates them into their own value system. Compliance can lead to internalisation if the individual is induced to behave in ways contrary to his beliefs under the minimum amount of inducement. This is predicted by cognitive dissonance theory, which is based on the premiss that people strive to achieve consistency between their beliefs and behaviour. This theory can be utilized to positively change behaviour (see Box 9.2).

The Ethics of Compliance

Regardless of the definition of compliance the term has connotations of authoritarianism and paternalism, the antipathy of modern nursing which aims to promote patient autonomy. The deontologist Immanuel Kant maintains that all human beings are unique, that every individual should be given the same respect regardless of whom they are, and that no one should be treated as a means to an end (Beauchamp and Childress, 1989). This means that each individual's rights should be respected and should not be sacrificed for the greater good. Taking Kant's argument to its logical conclusion there should be no compulsion for people to do what they do not want to do, and people should be permitted to be free.

However, can patients have the right to exercise their autonomy if it has detrimental effects on others? In matters of health, there is the danger that through exercising autonomy the patient can increase his morbidity and so make greater demands on the health service, depriving others of care. The utilitarian John Stuart Mill argues that it *is* justifiable to sacrifice an individual's freedom in order to promote the greatest happiness for the greatest number of people (Beauchamp and Childress, 1989). Certainly the government, in their reworking of the Patient's Charter (Department of Health, 1991), is making it clear that no person has rights without a corresponding level of responsibility. However, the Code of Conduct (UKCC, 1992) encourages nurses to take the view that people are an end in themselves and worthy of equal rights and treatment. Thus, nurses themselves must decide whether those equal rights have a limit (Jacob, 1994).

The Size of the Problem

The rate of compliance in patients suffering with chronic diseases is around the 50 per cent level (Cameron and Gregor, 1987; Kingsnorth and Wilkinson, 1996; Tettersell, 1993; Sackett and Haynes, 1976), which may suggest that the presence of a chronic disease can in itself contribute to non-compliance. The presence of chronic illness means that an individual has to alter their way of life, often to a monumental degree (Eddins, 1985). The person may feel stigmatised and find that their freedom and independence are limited (Cameron and Gregor, 1987; Tettersell, 1993; Kyngas and Barlow, 1995). For example, the patient with chronic renal failure on haemodialysis has his life constrained by the need for 2 or 3 times a week dialysis, as well as by severe fluid and dietary restrictions. Quality of life can be further impaired by the side effects of the disease for example bone demineralisation, pruritus and sexual impotence. This can lead on to depression, reduced self-esteem, hopelessness and helplessness; key factors in compliance (Charles 1996; House, 1996).

The Cost of Non-Compliance

The cost of non-compliance is difficult to measure. Ausburn (1981) assessed reasons for admission to medical wards among 205 patients and found that 20 per cent of admissions were probably, and a further 5 per cent were possibly, the result of medication non-compliance. Based on these findings, between one-tenth and one-quarter of medical inpatient beds may be occupied by patients who are in hospital due to non-compliance (Ley, 1988). This makes non-compliance very expensive. This is supported by the US Department of Health and Human Services, which estimated that the financial cost of non-compliance with ten common prescription drugs was $396–$792 million (Ley, 1988; see Box 9.3). On top of these financial considerations, there are also the costs to the patient and their family in terms of suffering and inconvenience.

Box 9.3 **Estimated costs of non-compliance with regimens for ten common drug classes**

Costings based on estimated 75 million prescriptions for ampicillins, benzodiazepines, cimetidine, clofibrate, digoxin, methoxsalen, propoxyphene, phenytoin, thiazides and warfarin. Assumed non-compliance rate of 40 per cent.

Source of cost	Estimated occurrence (%)	Estimated cost (1979–$ millions)
Unnecessary prescription refill	10.0–20.0	21.0–42.0
One additional visit to the doctor	5.0–10.0	22.5–45.0
One additional workday lost	5.0–10.0	67.5–135.0
Two additional workdays lost	5.0–10.0	135.0–270.0
1 days hospitalisation	0.25–0.5	18.75–37.5
2 days hospitalisation	0.50–1.0	75.0–150.0
3 days hospitalisation	0.25–0.5	56.26–112.5
Total		396–792

Source: Ley, 1988, p. 67 printed by kind permission of the author.

Measuring Non-Compliance

A statistic of 50 per cent non-compliance sounds quite drastic, but it needs to be put into context. Compliance is difficult to measure and usually indirect methods are used for the purpose (see Box 9.4). These methods are open to inaccuracy and frequently overestimate non-compliance. Thus when reading studies that measure compliance it is important to consider the methods used, together with their advantages and disadvantages.

Compliance can be monitored directly by observing the patient taking their medication. This might be possible to use in a hospital setting, but it is too time-consuming for use in the community. Tuberculosis therapy is one of the few areas where direct observation is utilized to monitor drug compliance. A more simplistic approach is to ask the patient if they are compliant. This has the advantage of being easy to do, but many researchers question the validity of this method as the patient might deceive, forget, or indeed believe that they are complying when they are not. As a method of measuring compliance however, it correlates significantly with other measures of compliance (Ley, 1988) and it is useful for identifying non-compliers (Gordis, 1979). To be effective the patient must be asked about their compliance in a non-judgemental manner, that is do you have any problems with your medication, rather than, do you follow health advice?

This can be a problem, as the issue of compliance is value laden, with compliance being seen as good and non-compliance being seen as bad. This point is clearly illustrated by Kyngas and Barlow's study (1995) that examines the adolescent's perspective of type 1 diabetes mellitus. Many of the adolescents in the study felt that the strict treatment regimes were impossible to comply with, and the expectations of their parents and healthcare workers were

---

Box 9.4 **Commonly used methods for measuring compliance**

- Direct observation
- Patient's selfreport
- Pill and bottle counts
- Mechanical devices
- Blood and urine tests for drug, metabolite or marker
- Outcome of treatment, i.e. the progress of the illness or condition
- Clinician's judgement

unrealistic. However, they did not feel able to admit this to their parents and healthcare staff as they felt that they ran the risk of receiving negative responses for their failure to meet the health goals set, so they lied. The lying was used as a coping mechanism that was effective in making relationships with healthcare staff and family tolerable. As a result of this lying, effective communication between the diabetic and his carers became impossible.

A popular method of monitoring compliance, particularly drug compliance, is the pill and bottle count. It is simple to measure or count the amount of drugs left, but it does not tell you if the patient has actually taken the medication, nor whether they followed the dosing schedule. Furthermore it does not allow for the use of tablet 'diaries' in which drugs are set out for an entire week. Alternatively, mechanical devices can be utilized which record every time the bottle is opened. These provide an accurate assessment of the timing of doses, but bottle opening need not correlate with drugs taken.

A more objective and accurate approach is to utilize blood and urine tests for a drug, its metabolite or some marker. Continuous monitoring is not realistic, but a single sample can be utilized. However, if the patient takes the medication correctly for a few days before visiting the doctor, the results might suggest, incorrectly, high levels of compliance. This used to be the case when blood sugar levels were utilized to monitor compliance with a diabetic lifestyle. The development of a test for glycosylated haemoglobin means that more long-term compliance can be monitored. Use of blood and urine tests can be expensive and they are not very acceptable to patients.

The commonest method of monitoring compliance is to utilize the treatment outcome, that is the progress of the illness or condition. This is relatively easy to do, but it ignores individual differences in response to treatment. Also the outcome variable may not be very responsive to changes in compliance, or affected by factors other than compliance with prescribed treatment. Thus for example, a patient who is trying to lose weight may have lost a significant amount of weight due to an episode of diarrhoea, even though they have not changed their eating behaviours or adhered to their diet.

The final method of measuring compliance employs the clinician's judgement. This is generally believed to be of low validity (Ley, 1988; Gordis, 1979). However, while the clinician's judgement that is normally considered is the doctor's, it would be interesting to discover if nurses are equally as inaccurate in identifying which of their clients are non-compliant.

Why are Patients Non-Compliant?

Raynor (1991) identifies three reasons for non-compliance, namely deliberate non-compliance; the regimen being too complicated to comply with; and the patient having insufficient information to comply.

Deliberate Non-Compliance

Patients with chronic diseases may deliberately choose to be non-compliant for a variety of reasons. They may be misinformed and thus, for example, believe that incontinence is a normal part of the ageing process, or that leg ulcers are an inherited disorder. The result of this judgement is that they may perceive treatment as a waste of time. Conversely, Weintraub (1981, cited in Raynor 1992) coined the term 'intelligent non-compliance' where a patient correctly identifies that their treatment is incorrect. Kelly (1994) describes the case of a lady who was prescribed anti-hypertensives that made her feel unwell. She informed her doctor and the medication was changed repeatedly. The lady continued to feel unwell, eventually stopped taking her medication, and as a result felt much better. Further exploration revealed that she was in fact normotensive – her hypertension being 'white coat syndrome'. This highlights a major problem. The diagnosis of some disorders, particularly hypertension, is difficult and the choice of the best treatment is open to debate. If we are not positive of our diagnosis and the best form of treatment has not been agreed upon, can we insist upon compliance?

Deliberate non-compliance may occur because of poverty. A recent survey found that up to a third of respondents were failing to get a doctor's prescription because of the high cost, while more worrying, 21 per cent said they had made a decision not to consult their GP because they feared the prescription charges (Anon, 1996 and see Box 9.5). Another reason for deliberate non-compliance is the fear of side effects or dependency. A survey of 540 London patients found that 30 per cent of patients had serious worries about their medication, much of which was unwarranted. Diabetics for example worried that they might become addicted to their insulin, while asthmatics were concerned about the long-term effects of using steroid inhalants (Horne, 1997; Kiernan, 1996).

Box 9.5 **Survey results from Kidderminster Community Health Council (Anon, 1995)**

Of the 300 respondents

35% were failing to obtain a doctor's prescription because of high costs

21% did not consult their GP due to fears of prescription charges

51% said they were chronically sick, e.g. had asthma, Parkinson's, AIDS, but were not eligible for free prescriptions

---

Box 9.6 **The 'social ulcer'**

The term 'social ulcer' has been used in relation to elderly patients with leg ulcers who refuse to comply with treatment because the presence of their ulcer ensures social contact. Wise (1986, p. 49) carried out a small study (10 patients) examining this issue and concluded that the study results 'appear to point to a relationship between non-healing of an ulcer and social isolation'.

As Tettersell (1993) found in her study the side effects that discourage patients from taking their drugs, are not just the pharmacological ones. Forty-eight per cent of patients in her study stated that they were reluctant to use their inhalers in public due to the stigma and embarrassment of doing so, and that they would prefer to take tablets. Furthermore, patients may have a low trust of healthcare personnel, which discourages them from following healthcare advice (Meichenbaum and Turk, 1987), especially when different members of the multi-disciplinary team are giving them different messages.

This is particularly a problem in chronic disease management where the patients is being cared for by a variety of hospital and community personnel. Finally, a reason occasionally suggested for deliberate non-compliance is a vested interest in keeping symptoms, as illustrated by the so-called 'social ulcer' (see Box 9.6).

Regimen Too Complicated

In the case of chronic diseases, such as diabetes, asthma and renal failure, the prescribed regime may be too complicated to adhere to. Forgetfulness may certainly be a reason and this is not just a problem of the elderly. Poulton (1991) identifies that immediately after a consultation roughly 40 per cent of what is said is forgotten. This forgetfulness will become increasingly problematic as health care advice becomes more detailed and complex. However, sometimes it is just the case that the client cannot fit the regimen into their lifestyle. Ertl (1992) found that non-compliance with compression hosiery frequently was because the clients were too frail to put it them on.

Insufficient Information

The patient may not have enough information to comply. The problem may be that staff believe that they have given the requisite information but

---

Box 9.7 **Reasons for patient's inability to take in health education**

- Poor attention due to over anxious state
- Organic difficulty, e.g. deafness blindness
- Toxic confusional states
- Language barriers
- Abstract nature of the information

Box 9.8 **Reasons why patients are not given the information they want**

- Staff do not have the knowledge or skills to provide the information clearly
- Staff have insufficient time to communicate
- Staff believe that patients do not want to know
- Staff believe that someone else has told the patient what they need to know
- Patient is reticent in asking questions

the patient has not taken it in for a variety of reasons (see Box 9.7). Alternatively, staff may not have given the patient all the information needed due to time constraints or incorrect beliefs that patients do not want to know (see Box 9.8). It is frequently assumed that nurses make good health educators, but Tettersell (1993) maintains that this is not necessarily the case, as 25 per cent of the patients she studied who had had an explanation about asthma from a nurse claimed to not have understood all that they were told.

Healthcare personnel frequently assume that insufficient information is the main reason for patient non-compliance. However, Brown (1996) maintains that, in over 220 studies, lack of knowledge was not the primary reason for patient non-compliance, although she does give the reason. This means that, although giving patients information about their disease and its management is important, nurses are unlikely to be able to increase patient compliance by *just* giving more information, and overloading a patient with information can be demotivating (Parkin, 1997). Instead nurses need to also consider patients' skills, particularly coping skills, and attitudes.

Who is Non-Compliant?

A wealth of research has been carried out over the years in an attempt to identify the characteristics of non-compliant patients, so that healthcare resources can be targeted at them in order to promote their compliance. This has been less than successful and many studies have come up with contradictory results. In a review of the literature on compliance Haynes *et al.* (1979, cited in Ley, 1988) found that out of 100 plus patient characteristics, 13 diseases, 13 regimens and 49 physician–patient interaction characteristics studied, the majority showed no association with compliance. Exceptions to this generalisation included Becker's Health Belief Model variables see Figure 9.1. These include the influence of friends and family, compliance

Figure 9.1   The Health Belief Model

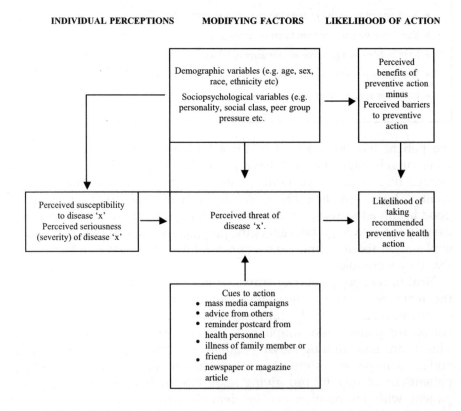

INDIVIDUAL PERCEPTIONS   MODIFYING FACTORS   LIKELIHOOD OF ACTION

Demographic variables (e.g. age, sex, race, ethnicity etc)

Sociopsychological variables (e.g. personality, social class, peer group pressure etc.

Perceived benefits of preventive action minus Perceived barriers to preventive action

Perceived susceptibility to disease 'x'
Perceived seriousness (severity) of disease 'x'

Perceived threat of disease 'x'.

Likelihood of taking recommended preventive health action

Cues to action
• mass media campaigns
• advice from others
• reminder postcard from health personnel
• illness of family member or
• friend
newspaper or magazine article

Source: J. King (1984b) 'Psychology in Nursing. The Health Belief Model' *Nursing Times* 80 (43): 53–5.

with other aspects of the regimen, duration of therapy, complexity of the reg-imen as assessed by the number of drugs or treatments involved, patients' satisfaction with their interaction with the therapist, patients' expectations being met by the therapist, and the level of supervision by the therapist.

Empowerment

Having discussed compliance at some length and the problems entailed, it is worth considering if compliance is what we actually want. A better term might be empowerment. Funnell *et al.* (1991) suggest 'patients are empowered when they have the knowledge, skills, attitudes and self-awareness necessary to influence their own behaviour and that of others in order to improve the quality of their lives'. An important focus of this definition is on quality rather than quantity. Healthcare personnel fre-quently concentrate on the latter, while the former is more important to patients. Cameron and Gregor (1987) suggest that whereas physical health is the priority for healthcare personnel, this is of secondary importance to patients whose priority is the pursuit of their personal goals. Healthcare personnel prescribe treatments to maintain or improve the patient's health, but the individual will not evaluate his regimen on whether or not it allows him to maintain a state of health.

Instead, the patient will judge the regimen on a social basis. This can lead to major problems if healthcare personnel and patients are looking at the problem from these very different perspectives, and this is recognized by Moore (1995, p. 71) who defines non-compliance as 'a lack of recogni-tion by the health care professional of the meaning of the regimen to the patient'. This definition reveals the need for negotiation between patient and nurse. It means that nurses need to make it clear to patients that they respect that the choice of changing their behaviour lies within the patient. All that nurses can do is ensure that patients are empowered to do so.

Promoting empowerment

In order to promote empowerment the first step is to develop a good nurse–patient relationship (Brown, 1997). This requires the nurse to have a non-judgemental attitude and to have a genuine concern for the patient. The nurse must also be prepared to compromise and to be honest. Without these traits a trusting relationship cannot develop, allowing the healthcare professional and client to work together in partnership to deal with the problems of coping with a chronic disease. Patients have to live with their diseases and so they become experts on their own condition, gleaning information from books, journals, and the Internet. Unless nurses accept patients' expertise, learn from them and discuss their care as one expert to another, they will not make much progress.

The relationship will benefit if the nurse is consistent in herself and if the client sees the same nurse each time. If the patient sees different nurses each time he comes to the practice, unless the nursing team have set very clear, detailed management protocols, there is the danger that the patient gets a slightly different message from each nurse. This might cause confusion, and cast doubt on the knowledge and skills of those advising and caring for him. This is demonstrated by Charles' (1996) study of leg ulcer healing. Of 114 patients with venous leg ulcers were treated with short stretch compression therapy – either by the leg ulcer team or by trained district nursing teams – the percentage of ulcers healed at three months was 81 per cent in the group managed by the leg ulcer team and 57 per cent in the group managed by the district nursing teams (see Box 9.9). In attempting to explain the differences in healing rates, Charles (1996) suggests that consistency of care may have been an important factor, as patients treated by the leg ulcer team were cared for by only two team members, while the patients treated by the district nurses had contact with a variety of staff.

Assessment

Having developed a relationship with the patient a comprehensive, holistic assessment needs to be carried out. Chronic illness is a long-term problem

---

Box 9.9 **Leg ulcer healing rates after three months**

Team	Number of Patients	Healed patients	Percentage healed
Leg ulcer team	47	38	81
Team A	3	2	67
Team B	21	11	52
Team C	14	9	64
Team D	20	11	55
Team E	9	5	55
Total	114	76	

(Adapted from Charles H., 1996) Developing a leg ulcer policy. *Professional Nurse* 11 (7): 475

Box 9.10   **Beliefs and attitudes**

- A belief is an expression of what we know, whereas an attitude is more of a value judgement, expressing what we feel. Attitudes can be discrepant with beliefs, as in the case of the person who knows smoking is dangerous but enjoys smoking.

Source: King, 1984a

---

and a good detailed initial assessment will pay dividends later. The assessment can utilise whichever model of nursing is being used by the practice, although Orem's Self Care Model is particularly useful. Having assessed the patient's usual self care parameters, the nurse should assess the patient's knowledge base. If the patient is confused or misinformed about his disease process, then he is not in a position to make an intelligent decision about whether to comply with his treatment. Also important is the patient's attitudes and beliefs about their disease (see Box 9.10). These are very difficult to assess, but are vital areas for consideration, as a patient will rarely follow advice that is incongruous with his existing beliefs (King, 1984b). Furthermore, King (1984a) identifies that for some physically dependent patients the only thing they have left are their attitudes and it can, therefore, be highly distressing to have them dismissed. Thus, beliefs and attitudes need to be explored with great care.

A detailed assessment of the patient's beliefs can be carried out utilizing the concepts of the Health Belief Model (see Figure 9.1). This model suggests that people are most likely to take preventive actions or comply with medical advice if they feel:

- concerned about their health and motivated to protect it
- threatened by their current behaviour
- change would be beneficial/have few adverse consequences
- competent to carry out change (Naidoo and Willis, 1995).

By eliciting information about the patient's health beliefs, the nurse can reinforce positive attitudes to health, to counter myths and negative attitudes (see Box 9.11).

Box 9.11   **Illustrative patient beliefs that can undermine treatment adherence**

- 'You only take medicine when you are ill and not when you feel better.'
- 'You need to give your body some rest from medicine once in a while or else your body becomes dependent on it or immune to it.'
- 'The medicine is so powerful that it should only be used for brief periods of time.'
- 'I miss the highs of my hypomanic life-style.'
- 'I don't feel the drug is doing anything.'
- 'I resent being controlled by drugs.'
- 'How will I know if I still need them if I keep taking pills?'
- 'What's the use of trying I knew I wouldn't be able to stay in control. Nothing I do seems to help.'

Source: and for further examples see Meichenbaum and Turk (1987)

Self Concept

Having completed a comprehensive assessment, Pfister-Minogue (1983) identifies that before a plan of care can be developed the patient must have accepted his disease and have a positive self concept. In listening to the patient's story the nurse may become aware that the patient is expressing, verbally or non-verbally, strong feelings such as anger, confusion, embarrassment, or despair in relation to living with his disease. Reflecting on these feelings can be essential in encouraging patients to come to terms with their condition. If the patient is still in denial over his diagnosis then it is impossible to produce a plan of care in partnership. You as the nurse may be able to do things to the patient, but not with the patient. It may be necessary to act in this way in the short term, for example administering the patient's insulin injections, but it is not a satisfactory solution.

The patient can be helped to accept his disease and develop a positive self concept, that is a belief that he can become master of his disease, through a variety of supportive strategies on the part of the nurse. Thus you can encourage the patient to verbalise his feelings and assist him to appreciate that his feelings of anger, depression and frustration are normal. Putting him in contact with a self support group may help this process. The patient may also be helped if the rest of the family can be encouraged to rally round and for a short time decrease the demands made on the patient, so that he has the energy to deal with his disease and the problems it entails. The patient should also be encouraged to focus on his strengths in order to promote positive self esteem.

Setting achievable goals

Once the patient is ready the nurse can then work with the patient to develop the self care behaviours to allow him to deal with his chronic disease in a positive way. One of the essential elements of the approach is to be specific. Thus, the patient should not be advised to lose weight, but should be told that they need to lose 12 kg. How the patient achieves this goal needs to be negotiated. He might prefer to alter his diet, or to alter his exercise pattern, or both. However, the plan must be individualised. So, rather than recommending a blanket reduction in fats and increase in vegetables, by carefully reviewing the patient's diet with him, and perhaps his wife, it may be possible to make painless minor changes which will bring about the desired response without requiring the patient to make major changes to his lifestyle.

If the goals are achievable then the patient is more likely to succeed, and success serves as an excellent reinforcement to carry on. The use of reinforcement and positive feedback will help, especially in the initial stages, to promote behaviour change. The nurse can give this feedback by perhaps monitoring the patient's progress through weekly weighing and drawing a graph to enable him to see his progress. His family and friends can also encourage and motivate him by giving praise, or by more concrete reinforcements such as trips out or presents. Again as part of the negotiation process the patient's personality should be taken into account, as some people progress better alone, and others do better by joining support groups such as Weight Watchers.

Success?

The result of the action plan may be that the patient changes his behaviour and adjusts positively to coping with his disease. Alternatively the patient verbally states that he wants to change his behaviour, but he does not seem to be able to be successful. In that case it is necessary to employ alternative or additional change strategies to achieve success.

The third possibility is that the patient refuses to change his behaviour and to comply with the recommended health strategies. If he understands his health problem, recognises that changing his behaviour might benefit his health, and recognises and accepts the implications of not changing his lifestyle, then the nurse *must* respect his choice. As a professional you are charged by the Code of Conduct (UKCC, 1992) to recognise the rights of the individual – you have to respect his decision.

Follow-up

This however is not the end of compliance promotion, or empowerment. It is common to start out with good intentions and then to falter along the way. By maintaining frequent follow-up appointments the nurse can help the patient with problems as they materialise, especially when there are lifestyle changes such as changing schools or job, getting married or having a baby. Also follow-up should not just be made available to patients that progress well or not so well, it should also be offered to patients who initially refused to change. As their life situation changes they may well be prepared to reconsider health changes, and the nurse needs to be prepared to help them as and when appropriate.

Conclusion

The intrinsic value judgement inherent in the term 'compliant' makes it unsuitable for use in present day nursing. If patients are to be involved as equal or even senior partners in decisions about their health then nurses can only act as expert advisers. Our aim must be to empower the patient so that they can take control of and responsibility for their own lives and make informed choices about their health and lifestyle.

10

Hypertension-risks and Detection

JENNY KELLY

What is Blood Pressure and How is it Controlled?

Blood pressure is the force exerted by the blood against a unit area of the blood vessel wall, and is dependent upon the cardiac output and the peripheral resistance (see Box 10.1). Maintenance of blood pressure is a homeostatic process involving neural and hormonal controls. Baroreceptors in the aortic arch and carotid bodies monitor the degree of stretch of the vessel walls and transmit this information to the cardiac and vasomotor centres in the medulla oblongata. If the blood pressure is low, signals are sent via the cardiac acceleratory centre and the sympathetic nervous system to the sino-atrial and atrio-ventricular nodes of the heart, causing the heart rate to increase. The vasomotor centre also sends nervous impulses to the smooth muscle of the arterial and venous vessels, causing the muscle to contract. Contraction of the arterial vessels increase peripheral resistance, while contraction of the venous smooth muscle increases venous return, and hence stroke volume and cardiac output (see Figure 10.1). When

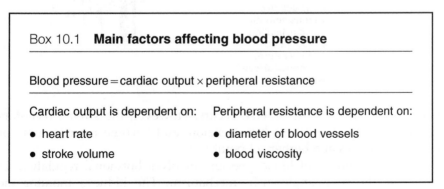

Box 10.1 **Main factors affecting blood pressure**

Blood pressure = cardiac output × peripheral resistance

Cardiac output is dependent on: Peripheral resistance is dependent on:

- heart rate
- stroke volume

- diameter of blood vessels
- blood viscosity

Figure 10.1   Homeostatic control of low blood pressure

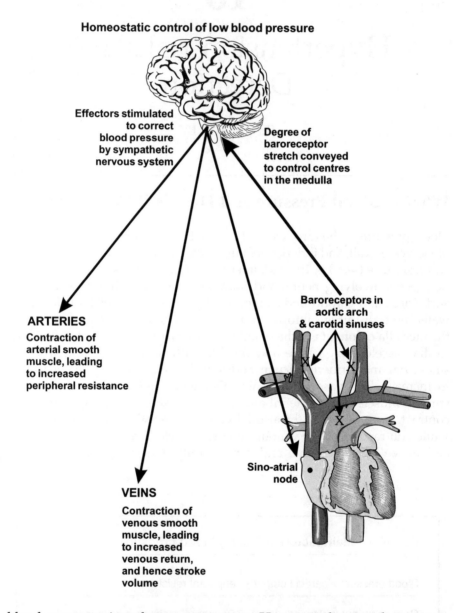

Homeostatic control of low blood pressure

Effectors stimulated to correct blood pressure by sympathetic nervous system

Degree of baroreceptor stretch conveyed to control centres in the medulla

ARTERIES

Contraction of arterial smooth muscle, leading to increased peripheral resistance

Baroreceptors in aortic arch & carotid sinuses

Sino-atrial node

VEINS

Contraction of venous smooth muscle, leading to increased venous return, and hence stroke volume

blood pressure rises the reverse occurs. However, the stretch receptors appear to adapt in chronic hypertension, and become reset to monitor pressure changes at a higher set point.

Long-term control of blood pressure involves hormonal regulation, in particular the renin-angiotensin mechanism. The kidneys monitor the pressure in the afferent arterioles supplying the glomeruli, as well as monitoring the osmolarity in the distal convoluted tubule of the nephrons. If either the pressure or osmolarity falls, the cells of the juxtaglomerular apparatus release the enzyme renin. This acts on the plasma protein angiotensinogen, cleaving it to form angiotensin I, which in turn is metabolised by angiotensin-converting enzyme (ACE) to form angiotensin II. Angiotensin II, which is a potent pressor substance, has a direct vasoconstrictor action on the vascular smooth muscle of the arterioles and arteries, but less action on the venous system. Angiotensin II also stimulates the adrenal cortex to release the hormone aldosterone, which causes the renal tubules to increase their re-absorption of sodium ions from the filtrate. This is accompanied by water re-absorption, leading to increased blood volume and increased systemic blood pressure (see Figure 10.2).

Figure 10.2   The renin-angiotensin system

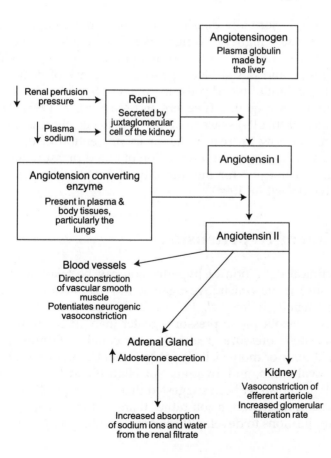

Other hormones also play a role in blood pressure control. The catecholamines – adrenaline and noradrenaline – which are produced as part of the 'fight or flight' response, increase blood pressure by increasing both cardiac output and peripheral resistance. Antidiuretic hormone (ADH), produced by the hypothalamus, stimulates the kidneys to conserve water, which helps to maintain blood pressure. When blood pressure is dangerously low ADH is released in large amounts and helps to restore arterial pressure by causing intense vasoconstriction. Cortisol, one of the hormones of the adrenal medulla, also plays a role by making blood vessels more sensitive to vasoconstrictive substances, as well as by causing the kidney to conserve salt and water. Atrial natriuretic peptides, produced by the atria of the heart, promote a reduction in blood volume and blood pressure by reducing renin and aldosterone secretion, stimulating the kidney to excrete more salt and water, and causing a general vasodilatation (Marshall, 1990).

Epidemiology of Hypertension

Blood pressure is normally distributed in the general population, with a slight skew towards higher readings. There is no evidence of a sub-group of hypertensives distinct from normotensives, and no dividing line between normal and raised blood pressure. The risk of death is directly related to the height of blood pressure, making hypertension a disease of quantity rather than quality (Beevers and MacGregor, 1995). This makes hypertension a difficult disease to define and, hence, there is much debate as to when and how to treat it. As far as prevention of disease is concerned, the aim should be for a reduction of blood pressure for the whole population and not just for the minority of people who are labelled as hypertensive (Whelton, 1994).

Definition of Hypertension

The best clinical definition of hypertension can be taken as the level of blood pressure above which investigation and treatment is of proven benefit to the patient (Grimley *et al.*, 1971). Based on our present state of knowledge this is a systolic blood pressure greater than, or equal to, 140 mmHg and/or a diastolic pressure greater than, or equal to, 90 mmHg, which is confirmed at three or more visits (Joint National Committee on Prevention, Detection, Evaluation, and Treatment of High Blood Pressure, 1997) (see Box 10.2). It has however been suggested that in younger clients it might be easier to treat mild hypertension rather than wait for severe hypertension and its complications to develop (Dickerson and Brown, 1995).

Box 10.2	**Classification of blood pressure for adults aged 18 years or older**

Category	Systolic BP (mmHg)	Diastolic BP (mmHg)
Normal	<130	<85
High normal	130–139	85–89
Hypertension		
• Stage 1	140–159	90–99
• Stage 2	160–179	100–109
• Stage 3	>=180	>=110

Source: based on the recommendations of the Sixth Joint National Committee on Prevention, Detection, Evaluation, and Treatment of High Blood Pressure (1997).

Essential Hypertension

Primary, or essential hypertension is elevation of blood pressure with no apparent cause. It accounts for over 90 per cent of cases and is usually seen after the age of 40 (Stevens and Lowe, 1995). The disease results from an interaction between genetic predisposition and a variety of risk factors, which are discussed below. How the risk factors operate is not known. It has been suggested that essential hypertension may result from a primary defect in renal sodium excretion, possibly combined with abnormalities in sodium or calcium transport in other cells. Any defect in sodium or calcium transport which leads to a rise in calcium levels in vascular smooth muscle would increase vascular tone, and hence blood pressure (Lakhani *et al.*, 1993). Vascular tone would also be affected by alteration in the level of the mediators listed in Box 10.3.

An alternative explanation, questions whether the morphological changes seen in arteriosclerotic arterioles are secondary to hypertension, or whether they are the cause. Small changes in the radius of a blood vessel will produce large changes in resistance. It is suggested that arterioles may initially constrict in response to a reversible vasoconstrictor but that they undergo remodelling with a permanent reduction in lumen size with chronic stimulation (Lakhani *et al.*, 1993). This is only speculation, but it is interesting to note that vasoconstrictors, such as adrenaline, also promote smooth muscle growth, and growth factors, such as platelet derived growth factor, can cause vasoconstriction.

Box 10.3 **Chemical mediators that effect vascular tone**

Constrictor	Dilators
• Angiotensin II	• Atrial natriuretic peptides
• Catecholamines, e.g. adrenaline	• Endothelium-derived relaxing factor
• Endothelin I	• Kinins
• Leukotrienes	• Nitric oxide
• Thromboxane	• Platelet activating factor
	• Prostaglandins

A third theory is that hypertension occurs as a repercussion of infection with *Chlamydia pneumoniae*. This is not as strange as it sounds considering that it is now accepted that stomach ulcers are usually the consequence of infection with another bacteria, *Helicobacter pylorii*. The evidence for this theory is a study by Cook *et al.* (1998) that found that 35 per cent of 123 patients with hypertension were infected with *Chlamydia pneumoniae* compared with 17.9 per cent of 123 matched normotensives. Cook suggests that *Chlamydia* causes inflammation of the blood vessels, which raises the blood pressure, leading in turn to atherosclerosis.

Risk Factors

Many factors have been associated with blood pressure levels in epidemiological surveys, and their relevance is open to considerable debate. Multiple risk factors have a synergistic effect on the chances of developing arterial complications (Beevers and MacGregor, 1995) and, hence, knowledge of these risk factors can be utilized in advising clients about lifestyle modifications (see Box 10.4).

Age

Most surveys demonstrate that systolic blood pressure tends to rise progressively throughout childhood, adolescence and adulthood to reach an average value of about 140 mmHg by the seventh or eighth decade (Whelton, 1994). However, studies of non-Westernised rural populations

---

Box 10.4   **Lifestyle modifications recommended by the British Hypertension Society**

Modifications for lowering blood pressure:

1. Reduction in total energy intake to achieve ideal body weight.

2. Avoidance of excessive alcohol intake (recommend <21 units per week in men and <14 units per week in women).

3. Reduction in salt intake by eliminating the use of table salt, reducing the use of salt when preparing food and avoiding excessively salty foods.

4. Regular physical exercise.

5. Increase fruit and vegetable consumption.

6. Decrease total fat and saturated fat intake.

Modifications to minimize cardiovascular disease:

1. Stop smoking.

2. Increase oily fish consumption.

3. Decrease total fat intake.

4. Replace saturated fat with polyunsaturated and monosaturated fats.

5. Avoidance of foods with high animal (saturated) fat and cholesterol content.

6. Regular physical exercise.

Source: Sever *et al.*, 1993.

---

have shown that hypertension is unknown in these groups, and that the trend of increasing blood pressure with age does not occur (Whelton, 1994). This indicates that the age-related changes are not a biological necessity. Furthermore, when the members of a rural population adopt a Western lifestyle they acquire a predisposition to age-related increases in blood pressure (Carvalho *et al.*, 1989; He *et al.*, 1991), suggesting that these changes are a result of lifestyle.

Alcohol Consumption

A link between increasing alcohol intake and hypertension has been shown in almost all of 50 cross-sectional and ten prospective population studies (Klatsky, 1995). For example a major study of 83 947 men and women found that regular intake of three or more drinks of alcohol a day was a risk factor for hypertension independent of age, sex, race, smoking, coffee use, former 'heavy' drinking, educational attainment and adiposity (Klatsky *et al.*, 1977).

White men and women reporting six or more drinks per day had a doubled prevalence of hypertension (↑160/95). In a randomised controlled crossover study of 44 men with treated essential hypertension, a reduction in weekly alcohol intake from 452 ml to 64 ml was associated with a fall in blood pressure of 5/3 mmHg in three weeks, independent of changes in weight (Puddey *et al.*, 1987). Conversely, small amounts of alcohol have been shown to be protective against coronary artery disease and ischaemic strokes, hence the J-shaped graph that relates deaths from all causes to alcohol consumption (Klatsky, 1995).

It has been suggested that the protective effect of wine is the result of a natural chemical – resveratol – which is found in grape skins, and which, based on its structure, acts like oestrogen (Boyce, 1998).

Diet

Epidemiological studies show that the prevalence of hypertension in a population is correlated with salt intake (Carvalho *et al.*, 1989), while animal experiments show that high salt intake will produce hypertension in most species. The importance of salt intake as a risk factor is supported by a rigorous analysis of 23 randomly controlled trials. This showed that a 100 mmol a day reduction in sodium intake was associated with a decline of 5.7/2.7 mmHg in hypertensive subjects, and 2.2/1.3 mmHg in normotensive individuals (Cutler *et al.*, 1991).

However, diets that are high in sodium are usually low in potassium, and potassium supplements have been shown to ameliorate the effects of hypertension in animals. A recent meta-analysis of 33 trials, involving 2609 subjects, demonstrated a significant reduction in mean systolic and diastolic pressures, of 3.11 g and 1.97 mmHg respectively, in those subjects receiving potassium supplementation (Whelton *et al.*, 1997). The effects of supplementation appeared to be enhanced in studies in which subjects had a high sodium intake. Other cations under investigation are calcium and magnesium, as deficiency in both have been implicated in the development of hypertension (Altura and Altura, 1995; McGee *et al.*, 1992).

Fat people have higher blood pressure than thin people (Beevers and MacGregor, 1995). However, a confounding factor here is that there is a greater error when measuring blood pressure in obese arms (see Box 10.5), such that the greater the arm size the greater the error. Nevertheless, the Intersalt study of 10 079 men and women aged between 20 and 59 (sampled from 52 communities world-wide) showed that body mass index, of all measured characteristics except age, had the strongest and most consistent correlation with blood pressure (Intersalt Cooperative Research Group, 1988). Individuals with central or upper body obesity, as indicated by a higher waist-to-hip ratio, are particularly likely to have a raised blood pressure (Alderman, 1994). Weight reduction lowers blood pressure, and Reisin *et al.* (1978) showed that with sodium and potassium intake held constant, a weight loss of about 5 kg was associated with a decline of 5.4/2.4 mmHg.

There is also evidence that people with diets high in animal fats have higher blood pressures than those who eat unsaturated fats. A change from a Mediterranean diet to one rich in saturated fats causes an increase in blood pressure (McGee *et al.*, 1992).

Early Life Experiences

It has been suggested that adverse environmental conditions during critical periods of development in foetal life and infancy predisposes an individual to hypertension. Several cohort studies have shown an inverse relationship between weight, measured at birth or one year, and adult levels of blood pressure. Furthermore, Barker *et al.* (1990) demonstrated an independent positive relationship between placental weight and adult blood pressure in both men and women, such that highest blood pressures occurred in those who had been, at term, small babies with large placentas. Barker *et al.* (1990) speculate that the discordance between placental and foetal size leads to circulatory adaptation in the foetus, altered arterial structure in the child, and hypertension in the adult.

This suggests that prevention of hypertension would, therefore, depend on improving the nutrition and health of mothers. However, others have questioned the causality of these relationships, especially as immigrants assume the disease pattern of their new home, which emphasizes the importance of adult, rather than childhood, environments (Whelton, 1994).

Genetic Factors

The ability to produce animal models of hypertension by selective breeding provides strong evidence that genetic factors are important determinants of high blood pressure (Kurtz, 1994). Twin studies, together with studies comparing blood pressure of adopted and natural children of the same parents also support a genetic component to the disease (McGee *et al.*, 1992). The unimodal distribution of blood pressure in human populations suggests it is a polygenic trait (Harrap, 1994) involving perhaps as many as 10 or 15 genes.

However, the fact that migration studies demonstrate that the migrants' blood pressure mirrors that of the endogenous population, suggests that environmental factors are more important than genetic factors as determinants of blood pressure (He *et al.*, 1991).

Physical Activity

Dynamic exercise raises blood pressure and isometric exercise raises it a lot. Despite this people who take a lot of exercise are healthier and may have lower blood pressures than those who take none. This may be because they are thinner and tend to have more sensible dietary, drinking and smoking habits. Also, after exercise blood pressure falls and people who take regular exercise may, therefore, have lower pressures for longer periods of the day (Beevers and MacGregor, 1995).

Race

In the USA, national surveys have demonstrated that hypertension is at least twice as prevalent in the Afro-Caribbean as in the Caucasian population, and that it has a worse prognosis. One explanation is that the differences between Afro-Caribbeans and Caucasians are partially the result of genetics, with high renin levels, enhanced sodium sensitivity and increased adrenergic reactivity to stress having the strongest experimental support (Kaplan, 1994). Hypertensive Afro-Caribbean men have a death rate about six times that of Caucasian men with the same level of blood pressure (McGee *et al.*, 1992), as they have more ventricular hypertrophy and nephrosclerosis than do Caucasians with similar degrees of hypertension (Kaplan, 1994). However, Cooper *et al.*'s (1999) study of Africans, as well as people of African descent living in the Caribbean and USA, demonstrated a dramatic drop in hypertension from the USA across the Atlantic to Africa, suggesting that the problem is largely one of modern lifestyle rather than genetics. It is interesting to note that if Cook's theory (1998) that hypertension is a repercussion of infection with *Chlamydia pneumoniae* is correct, this may explain the apparent racial difference, because in his study *Chlamydial* infection was found to be twice as high in blacks as in whites.

Gender

Early in life there is little evidence of a difference in blood pressure between the sexes, but beginning in adolescence men tend to display a higher average level. Later in life the difference narrows and the pattern is often reversed. This change partly reflects the premature deaths of men with high blood pressure (Whelton, 1994). Overall, mortality rates for men are 1.5 to 2 times that of women (McGee *et al.*, 1992).

Smoking

Cigarette smoking increases the risk of developing malignant hypertension in hypertensive patients. However, of much greater importance is its role as a major risk factor in ischaemic heart disease, and the other complications of atheroma (McGee *et al.*, 1992).

Socio-Economic status

In many studies socio-economic status has been closely associated with average levels of blood pressure, with those in the lower classes having higher blood pressures. For example in the Whitehall Study of British civil servants the average value for systolic pressure varied from 133.7 mmHg in the highest grade of employment to 139.9 mmHg in the lowest (Whelton, 1994). It has been suggested that this correlation arises from the fact that those of higher socio-economic status have more control over their lives and are, therefore, less stressed. Diet is also a confounding factor.

Stress

Urban populations have higher blood pressures than rural populations and the adverse effects of urban living are confirmed by the rise in blood pressure of rural populations migrating to the cities. These and similar studies, including experiments in which animals are subject to a chronically stressful environment, suggest the effect of stress (McGee *et al.*, 1992). However, there remains considerable doubt as to whether chronic stress does raise blood pressure, as investigations of environmental stress are confounded by other social factors including poverty, dietary fats, calorie, electrolyte and alcohol intake, and cigarette smoking (Beevers and MacGregor, 1995). Furthermore, stress is very difficult to measure, especially as what might be stressful for one person is not for another.

Secondary Hypertension

Secondary hypertension, where there is an identifiable cause for the raised blood pressure, accounts for around 10 per cent of cases of hypertension.

The main cause is renal disease, which may be due to stenosis of one of the renal arteries by atherosclerosis or a mechanical factor. As a result the stenosis blood pressure entering the kidney is low. The kidney responds as if this is the state in the rest of the body and attempts to raise the blood pressure by releasing renin, resulting in increased levels of angiotensin II.

Hypertension is also a feature of diffuse renal diseases such as glomerulonephritis and pyelonephritis. The hypertension is transient in the initial acute phase of glomerular disease, but is permanent in chronic renal disease. The prevalence of renovascular disease is less than 1 per cent in the general population of hypertensives, but accounts for up to 40 per cent of patients referred to hypertension clinics (Derkx and Schalekamp, 1994). Other causes of secondary hypertension include:

- phaeochromocytoma – an adrenaline secreting tumour of the adrenal medulla

- adrenal cortical diseases such as Cushing's and Conn's syndromes in which there is excess production of glucocorticoids and mineralcorticoids (see Gordon, 1994)

- co-arction of aorta – a congenital malformation in which there is increased peripheral resistance due to a structural narrowing of the aorta; the hypertension is localised to the arterial system proximal to the co-arction, that is the arms, head and neck

- pre-eclampsia – in one explanation the ischaemic placenta produces renin leading to vasoconstriction

- neurogenic – as caused by raised intracranial pressure, in for example head injury.

Benign or Malignant

Depending on the clinical course of the disease both primary and secondary hypertension can be classified into two types, benign and malignant. In the case of the former, there is a stable elevation of blood pressure over many years and few clinical symptoms. However, with malignant hypertension, which only affects 5 per cent of hypertensives, elevation is severe and if untreated is usually fatal in less than a year (Lindop, 1992).

Complications of Hypertension

Hypertension itself is usually asymptomatic, consequently people are not aware that they have a problem and so do not seek help. However, a

---

Box 10.5 **Complications of hypertension**

Organ	Diseases
Heart	Left ventricular hypertrophy and failure, angina pectoris, cardiac arrhythmias, myocardial infarction
Blood vessels	Atherosclerosis and aneurysm formation
Lungs	Pulmonary oedema due to left ventricular failure
Brain	Microaneurysms, cerebral thrombosis, intracerebral haemorrhage
Kidneys	Ischaemic cortical damage, renal failure
Eyes	Retinopathy, blindness
Lung, colon, kidney, etc.	? Cancer (see Hamet, 1996)

---

sustained increase in blood pressure over a period of time has deleterious effects on the organs of the body, in particular the cardiovascular system and the brain (see Box 10.5).

As far as the cardiovascular system is concerned, atheroma formation is the main problem. However, elevated blood pressure by itself does not induce atherosclerosis. Instead hypertension results in altered arterial structure and function and abnormal blood flow patterns, which in the presence of other risk factors, such as hypercholesteraemia, accelerates the progression of atherosclerosis (Hamel and Oberle, 1996). Atherosclerosis in turn leads to narrowing of the arteries, peripheral vascular disease, ischaemic heart disease and emboli formation. Aneurysms are also more common in hypertensive patients, and there is increased risk of dissection.

About 50 per cent of patients with moderate hypertension have left ventricular hypertrophy. If this complication is present, there is a threefold increase in the patient's risk of developing intermittent claudication, a four-fold increase in the risk of a heart attack and a twelve-fold increase in the risk of a stroke, compared with a patient with a similar blood pressure but no hypertrophy (Beevers and MacGregor, 1995). For this reason the routine use of electrocardiogram, which can identify hypertrophy, in a new hypertensive patient is a powerful predictor of outcome. Nowadays echocardiography is valuable to confirm or refute the presence of left ventricular hypertrophy (BHS, 1999). The Joint British Societies Coronary Risk Prediction Chart can also be used for estimating coronary heart disease risk for individuals who have not developed symptomatic coronary heart disease or other major atherosclerotic disease (see Ramsay *et al.*, 1999).

Hypertension is the single most important risk factor for cerebrovascular disease. It causes adaptive changes in the cerebral circulation leading to transient cerebral ischaemic attacks and strokes. Hypertension may also cause headaches and occasionally acute hypertensive encephalopathy (Strandgaard and Paulson, 1994).

How Should we Screen for Hypertension?

As hypertension is a problem for such a large proportion of the population, it is arguable that every adult (18 years or older) should be screened. The American Academy of Family Physicians suggests that blood pressure should be measured at every visit, with a minimum frequency of two yearly, while the American College of Physicians recommends that blood pressure should be measured every one to two years. Normotensive patients should have blood pressure measurements at least yearly if they:

- have a diastolic pressure between 85 and 89 mmHg
- have an Afro-Caribbean heritage
- are moderately obese
- have a first-degree relative with hypertension
- have a personal history of hypertension (Anon, 1996).

Hypertension can only be identified by measurement of blood pressure. However, although the process of measuring blood pressure is frequently performed, and is regarded by medical and nursing personnel as a simple task (O'Brien and Davison, 1994), it is frequently carried out incorrectly (Edwards, 1997). A study by Kemp *et al.* (1993) of 100 nurses found that 40 per cent claimed to have had no formal training in the technique, while 50 per cent admitted to occasional estimation of systolic pressure, diastolic, or both. These findings are of great concern as the use of an incorrect or careless technique can lead to wrong diagnosis which may result in unnecessary or inappropriate treatment and follow up (Petrie *et al.*, 1986).

Blood pressure is measured using a sphygmomanometer. This can be mercury, aneroid or electronic, each of which has its advantages and disadvantages (see Box 10.6). The correct procedure for blood pressure measurement is outlined in Box 10.7, while Box 10.8 highlights some of the main areas of possible inaccuracy which the competent practitioner needs to be aware of and guard against. It has been argued that the best person to measure a patient's blood pressure is a nurse as it is likely to be lower than when it is measured by a doctor, and also closer to the patient's day time average level of blood pressure (Pickering, 1994). The rationale behind

---

Box 10.6 **Types of sphygmomanometer**

Mercury sphygmomanometer – measures cuff pressure by means of a vertical column of mercury

Advantages:	Disadvantages:
• accurate	• not as portable as the aneroid
• easy to read	• contains poisonous mercury
• no moving parts to be damaged	• must be serviced every 6–12 months

Aneroid sphygmomanometer – measures cuff pressure by means of a spring-operated gauge

Advantages:	Disadvantages:
• light, compact and easily portable	• loses its accuracy with time, leading to falsely low readings
• relatively small dial	• spring and internal moving parts may be damaged
	• must be checked and calibrated every 6–12 months
	• flickering dial makes reading difficult

Electronic sphygmomanometer – either detects Korotcofvt Sounds by means of a Microphone, or detects arteral blood flow by ultrasonography or oscillometry

Advantages:	Disadvantages:
• At least as accurate as a mercury sphygmomanometer	• Can cause pain if the cuff is inflated too tightly
• Easy to read.	• May not record accurate readings in patients with atrial fibrillation.

---

this is that nurses are seen as more approachable by patients, so 'white-coat' hypertension is less of a problem. This is particularly important as among hypertensives the prevalence of 'white-coat' syndrome is between 20 and 35 per cent (Staessen *et al.*, 1997). Another possible solution to this problem is self-monitoring by the patient. This has the advantages that distortion produced by the 'white-coat' effect is eliminated and that multiple readings can be taken over long periods. The main problem is the greater chance for observer error (Pickering, 1994, see Box 10.9).

Another alternative is the use of ambulatory pressure measurement, which has been shown to correlate more closely with the extent of target

Box 10.7   **How to take an accurate blood pressure**

1. The patient has not eaten, exercised or smoked for at least half an hour prior to the blood pressure being taken, and has an empty bladder.

2. The procedure is explained to the patient, so as to reduce anxiety.

3. The patient is sitting or lying comfortably in a warm, quiet environment with his arm resting at heart level on a pillow – the antecubital fossa is level with the fourth intercostal space.

4. The patient has been lying or sitting for at least 3 minutes, or standing for at least 1 minute, prior to blood pressure measurement.

5. The appropriate sized bladder is used (see Box 10.8) with the centre of the bladder over the brachial artery.

6. The cuff is applied high enough up the arm to allow a 2–3 cm gap between it and the antecubital fossa.

7. The sphygmomanometer is placed on a flat surface, at eye level, with the mercury level at zero.

8. The brachial artery is located by palpation.

9. The cuff is inflated while palpating the radial pulse, until the pulse can no longer be felt. The valve is released and the cuff let down.

10. The stethoscope is placed over the brachial artery taking care not to use too much pressure as this lowers the diastolic reading.

11. The cuff is inflated to a maximum pressure of 20–30 mmHg higher than that required to ablate the radial pulse. This allows the blood pressure to be measured while causing minimal discomfort to the patient.

12. The valve is released slowly and gently, allowing the cuff to deflate at a rate of 2 mmHg per second or heart beat, while listening for the Korotkov sounds (Beevers and Macgregor, 1988).

13. The systolic pressure is noted at the onset of the first clear repetitive tapping sound (phase 1).

14. The diastolic pressure is recorded at the cessation of sound (phase 5), unless the recording is zero, in which case the muffling of sound (phase 4) should be used. If phase 4 is used, it should be documented on the chart.

15. Blood pressure should be measured to the nearest 2 mmHg.

16. Make two measurements at each visit (Ramsay *et al.*, 1999), allowing at least 2 minutes to elapse before re-inflating the cuff.

Box 10.8 **Cuff (bladder) sizes (Petrie *et al.*, 1986)**

The cuff consists of an inflatable bladder inside a cloth sheath. As long as the sheath wraps securely around the arm, its length is not important. However, the length and width of the inflatable bladder are critical.

Length of bladder:

- If too short, the blood pressure will be overestimated.

- It should be at least 80% of the midpoint* arm circumference.

- For normal adult arms a 35 cm bladder is strongly recommended.

- For heavily muscled or obese arms a bladder 42 cm long may be required.

- The bladder usually supplied is 23 cm. If used the centre of the bladder must be centred over the artery.

Width of bladder:

- To narrow a bladder leads to overestimation of blood pressure.

- It should be at least 40% of the arm circumference.

- In adults with lean, through to obese arms a cuff of 12–15 cm is recommended.

* Midpoint is defined as half the distance from acromion to olecranon (Draper, 1987)

Adapted from S. Edwards (1997) recording Blood Pressure. *Professional Nurse* Supplement 13 (2) S10.

---

organ damage than clinic pressure (Pickering, 1994). In a study by Staessen *et al.*, 1997, 419 patients, with untreated diastolic pressures averaging 95 mmHg or higher, were randomised to either ambulatory (ABP) or conventional blood pressure monitoring (CBP), and treatment with antihypertensives. The researchers found that by the end of the study more ABP patients had stopped antihypertensive treatment (26 per cent) than CBP patients (7.3 per cent), and fewer ABP patients had progressed to sustained multiple-drug treatment than CBP patients (27.2 per cent versus 42.7 per cent). Although ambulatory blood pressure monitoring is expensive, the study found that the savings in drugs and visits to the doctor offset the costs. Clinical situations in which ambulatory blood pressure monitoring may be useful are given in Box 10.10.

One of the main advantages of ambulatory blood pressure monitoring is that it gives multiple blood pressure readings on which to base the client's diagnosis, rather than just one. The use of multiple blood pressure

Box 10.9 **Potential sources of error in blood pressure measurement**

The patient

- fear, anxiety and pain can raise blood pressure
- if the patient is talking this may raise the pressure (Pickering, 1994)
- a recent meal in the elderly can lower pressure by 5–10 mmHg (Pickering, 1994)
- 'white coat syndrome' causes transient increase in blood pressure
- calcified/rigid arteries can give false, high readings
- Time of day – systolic blood pressure can be lower in the morning and higher in the evening
- in hypotension, there may be distal vasoconstriction, causing an under estimation of blood pressure
- obese arms – can lead to over estimation of blood pressure, in excess of 16 mmHg for diastolic readings (Draper, 1987).

Equipment

- incorrect cuff size (see Box 10.8)
- mercury level not at zero
- sphygmomanometer not at eye level
- equipment incorrectly calibrated; calibration should be checked at least six monthly (O'Brien and Davison, 1994). Conceicao *et al.* (1976) found that almost half the sphygmomanometers in teaching hospital had defects
- perished rubber tubing that allows air to leak out
- defective control valve making control difficult
- stethoscope in poor condition, with dirty, poorly fitting earpieces.

The observer

- lack of understanding/knowledge on how to perform the procedure correctly, e.g. position the sphygmomanometer at the same level as the patient's heart
- hearing or sight problems
- basing the present reading on the previous one
- digit preference – only recording readings divisible by 5.

Source: adapted from S. Edwards (1997) recording Blood Pressure, *Professional Nurse* Supplement 13 (2): S10.

Box 10.10 **Situations when automated non-invasive ambulatory blood pressure monitoring devices may be useful**

- 'White-coat' hypertension.
- Evaluation of drug resistance.
- Evaluation of nocturnal blood pressure changes.
- Episodic hypertension.
- Hypotensive symptoms associated with antihypertensive drugs or autonomic dysfunction.
- Carotid sinus syncope and pacemaker syndromes (together with electrocardiographic monitoring).

Source: based on the recommendations of the Sixth Joint National Committee on Prevention, Detection, Evaluation, and Treatment of High Blood Pressure (1997).

measurements is clearly supported by a study conducted by Pheley *et al.* (1995) which demonstrated that the use of multiple measurements resulted in 215 (78.2 per cent) of patients not starting antihypertensive therapy, who would have done so if their management had been based on one blood pressure measurement.

A study by Agrawal *et al.* (1996) suggests that blood pressure measurement could be augmented by qualitative microalbuminuria screening in the practice setting, to identify non-diabetic hypertensive patients at high risk of developing cardiovascular disease. Their study of 11 343 non-diabetic hypertensive patients demonstrated that qualitative measurement of microalbuminuria using an albumin-sensitive immunoassay test strip provided a good indication of patients with underlying cardiovascular disease. The British Hypertension Society (Sever *et al.*, 1993) states that urinalysis, measurement of serum electrolytes and of urea are essential for all hypertensive patients, while an electrocardiogram, measurement of blood glucose and serum lipids is also recommended. Once diastolic blood pressure is stabilised below 90 mmHg with treatment, three-monthly measurement of blood pressure is sufficient follow-up.

However, some patients are drug resistant, that is they have a diastolic blood pressure greater than 95 mmHg at three visits several weeks apart, despite treatment with two classes of antihypertensive drugs. These patients should be screened for renovascular disease (Derkx and Schalekamp, 1994).

Should we Screen for Hypertension?

Screening refers to the detection of presymptomatic abnormalities in a population (DHSS, 1977) and its main aim is to reduce mortality and morbidity from the disease. To be suitable for screening a disease should have four characteristics, namely:

- its prevalence is high
- it has a slow but progressive natural history
- its effects are major
- and early therapy gives better results than late therapy (Elwood, 1990).

The problem with hypertension is that it is a disease of quantity rather than quality. Thus the prevalence of the disease is open to debate depending on where it is arbitrarily decided to make the cut off. If the cut off point of 140/90 mmHg is used, then as indicated above approximately 50 million Americans (Anon, 1996) and 15 million people in the UK suffer from hypertension (Lakhani *et al.*, 1993, p. 109), making hypertension a very common problem.

Hypertension in most countries is age-related, with most surveys demonstrating a gradual rise in blood pressure throughout childhood, adolescence and adulthood. Thus as pathology is related to level of blood pressure, in the case of benign essential hypertension, it is true to say that the disease has a slow but progressive history.

The effects of hypertension are certainly major. Cardiovascular disease is the main cause of death in virtually all industrialised countries and hypertension is a major risk factor for this condition (Whelton, 1994). This is clearly supported by the results from pooling of data derived from 418 343 adults, aged 25–70 years, who were initially free of coronary heart disease, and who participated in nine prospective observational studies for an average of ten years follow-up (MacMahon *et al.*, 1990). The risk of coronary heart disease was nearly five times higher for those with the highest diastolic blood pressure (105 mmHg), compared with those with the lowest (76 mmHg). Risk of stroke was more than 10 times higher between the two groups. The data suggest that a 5–6 mmHg lower level of diastolic pressure is typically associated with a 20–25 per cent lower risk of coronary heart disease (Collins *et al.*, 1990). Barker *et al.* (1990) suggest that lowering the distribution of blood pressure among a population by 10 mmHg would correspond to a 30 per cent reduction in total attributable mortality. Furthermore, Linjer and Hansson (1997) suggest that the results of the studies investigating the value of antihypertensive treatment underestimate its true benefits.

So, the final question to ask is does early therapy give better results than late therapy? Certainly, treatment for hypertension is very effective and has contributed to a 57 per cent reduction in mortality from stroke and a 50 per cent reduction in mortality from coronary artery disease in the USA in the last 24 years (Anon, 1996). The benefits of antihypertensive therapy are greatest in those with the most marked elevations in blood pressure. However, even patients with mild hypertension benefit from treatment (Anon, 1996). Therefore, in theory the sooner hypertension is detected, the sooner the patient can benefit.

Unfortunately, the issue of screening is more complicated. Cochrane and Holland (1971) suggest, 'there is an ethical difference between everyday medical practice and screening. If a patient asks a medical practitioner for help, the doctor does the best he can. He is not responsible for defects in medical knowledge. If, however, the practitioner initiates screening procedures he is in a very different situation.' He should, in their view, 'have conclusive evidence that screening can alter the natural history of the disease in a significant proportion of those screened.' This means that he must first be sure of his diagnosis.

A major problem with screening for hypertension is the difficulty of measuring blood pressure correctly (see Box 10.7). Chatellier and Menard (1997) suggest that the order of magnitude of the error in measurement of blood pressure is 10 mmHg. This together with the 'white-coat' effect means that many patients who are not hypertensive could be treated inappropriately. As Box 10.11 indicates, the drugs used to treat hypertension have some unpleasant, if not lethal, side effects. According to a study carried out by Psaty *et al.* (1995), the use of short-acting calcium channel blockers to treat hypertension, especially in high doses, is associated with an increased risk of myocardial infarction. Thus, if nurses are going to be involved in screening for hypertension, they must be very sure of their technique for measuring blood pressure, and they must use multiple measurements to ensure that patients are not treated unnecessarily (Pheley *et al.*, 1995).

Screening and the Elderly

Most elderly people with hypertension have isolated systolic hypertension, defined as a systolic pressure greater than 140 mmHg and a diastolic pressure of less than 90 mmHg (Bennet, 1994). As with younger age groups the value of screening is supported by research, with recent large clinical trials showing that antihypertensive treatment in elderly patients is highly protective against stroke and myocardial infarction (Strandgaard and Paulson, 1994). The STOP trial, which studied 1627 men and women aged 70–84, demonstrated a significantly reduced number of deaths in the

Box 10.11   **Drugs used in the management of hypertension and their side effects**

Drug Group	Adverse effects
Diuretics, e.g. amiloride, bendroflurazide, hydrochlorothiazide	Increased urination, hypotension, hypokalaemia or hyperkalaemia depending on type, glucose intolerance in long-term use, hyperuricaemia, hypercalcaemia, sexual dysfunction, fatigue, levels of low density lipoproteins, decreased levels of high density lipoproteins
β-blockers, e.g. atenolol, bisoprolol	Bronchospasm, fatigue, lethargy, insomnia, nightmares, depression, lack of concentration, impotence, decreased exercise intolerance, postural hypotension, bradycardia
Centrally acting, e.g. minoxidil	Nausea, weight gain, hirsuitism
ACE inhibitors, e.g. captopril, enalapril, lisinopril	Dry persistent cough, rash, hyper kalaemia, acute renal failure, angioedema, hypotension, dizziness, fatigue, diarrhoea, headache
Calcium channel blockers, e.g. amlodipine, diltiazem, nifedipine, verapamil	Constipation, headaches, dizziness, hypotension, flushing, peripheral oedema, gingival hyperplasia, AV block, bradycardia or tachycardia depending on type, myocardial infarction
α-blockers, e.g. doxazosin, prazosin	Dizziness, headache, drowsiness, postural hypotension, blurred vision, insomnia
Angiotensin II receptor antagonists, e.g. candesartan, irbesartan, losartan, valsartan	Headache, back pain, dizziness, hypotension. Relatively new group of drugs so adverse effects not fully documented
Selective imidazoline receptor agonists, e.g. moxonidine	Dry mouth, somnolence, headache, and dizziness. Relatively new group of drugs so adverse effects not fully documented.

active treatment group compared with the placebo group (36 versus 63) (Dahlof *et al.*, 1991).

However, when screening the elderly a few modifications need to be made to the procedure. First, blood pressure readings are far more variable in the elderly, so more readings need to be taken before a diagnosis is made (Bennet, 1994). Second, blood pressure should be measured in both the sitting and standing position. This is because there is frequently (30 per cent in the NHANES II Survey (NHANES, 1986 cited Bennet, 1994)) a drop of 20 mmHg in standing blood pressure in patients with a sitting pressure of 160 mmHg. Standing blood pressure measurements should be used to guide treatment decisions. If standing blood pressure is not utilized to guide treatment decisions, there is a danger that the postural hypotension will be made worse, leading to falls and the serious consequences that they entail. More seriously inappropriate treatment of postural hypotension may lead to cerebral ischaemia and possibly dementia (Standgaard and Paulson, 1994).

The British Hypertension Society recommends treatment thresholds of 160 mmHg systolic, or 90 mmHg diastolic, or both, for elderly patients of 60–80 years (Sever *et al.*, 1993). However, not all elderly hypertensives should be treated. Account must be taken of the patient's overall medical condition. It may be better not to prescribe anti-hypertensive medication for the very sick or medically complicated (Medicines Resource Centre, 1993).

Conclusion

Hypertension is a major disease of Western populations. Measuring the patient's blood pressure in the clinic can easily screen it the condition. However, nurses must be sure that they have the skills and correctly working equipment to perform the assessment, and if they do not, they must take steps to remedy the situation.

11

Case Management of the Hypertensive Patient

SALLY QUILLIGAN

Introduction

High blood pressure is a symptom and not a disease. Persistently raised blood pressure will place a person at increased risk of stroke and is often indicative of underlying atherosclerosis – coronary heart disease. Coronary heart disease is a major health problem, causing 170 000 deaths annually. Thirty per cent of all male deaths and 23 per cent of female deaths are attributed to coronary heart disease. Coronary heart disease remains the major cause of death in the UK (Department of Health, 1994).

The 1990 GP contract saw the establishment of many hypertension and coronary heart disease clinics run by practice nurses. A survey by Jones (1995), however, suggested that of the three chronic disease management clinics – asthma, diabetes and hypertension – the latter was the area in which the practice nurses felt least autonomous. This almost certainly reflects the fact that until very recently there was no specialist training in this field. The value of the practice nurse's role in this area has, however, now been acknowledged. At the inaugural meeting of the REACH (Rational Evaluation and Choice in Hypertension (1998)) primary care group one of the key conclusions was that 'well trained practice nurses should be encouraged to assume greater ownership of hypertension'.

The following case study discussion aims to highlight the valuable role the practice nurse can play in the management of patients with hypertension and coronary heart disease. The framework for the discussion is based on the practice protocol, which was jointly drawn up by the GPs and the practice nurses. Throughout the discussion the emphasis is on patient education and patient involvement in all aspects of their care. The aim is to show that by working with these patients and taking time to develop a trusting relationship, it is possible to help them through adaptation to lifestyle changes including taking long-term medication.

James – a Case Study

James presents in a busy evening surgery. A colleague at work has recently been diagnosed as hypertensive and so he has decided he had better get his blood pressure checked. He appears very anxious. He has been added to your already busy evening surgery what initial action would you take? You should act to reassure him that it is sensible to have his blood pressure checked every three years even if it is normal.

While letting him sit comfortably, explain the procedure and position his arm comfortably level with his heart. After checking the bladder of the cuff covers 80 per cent of his arm fit the cuff. Make sure he is aware that the electronic monitor requires him not to talk while the reading is being recorded and that the cuff will feel very tight for approximately 30–40 seconds. At least 3 minutes after he first sat down record first blood pressure reading and repeat twice more at 5 minutes intervals.

The initial reading was 200/110 mmHg. Aware of his anxiety I decided to briefly assess his current situation. His notes were very thin and there was no significant past medical history. He was a 64-year-old, married man who was a non-smoker. He had worked as the Managing Director of a company that employed 46 people for 27 years, but as he was preparing for retirement had recently reduced his hours to a three-day week. He commented that he found this position very frustrating and was constantly finding that things were not being done as he expected them to be. As he talked, he began to relax, sitting more casually in the chair and crossing his legs. He volunteered his family history without being asked. His brother had died of a heart attack aged 45 and his father had suffered from severe angina from the age of 60. The second BP reading was 185/100 mmHg.

What factors might have influenced his blood pressure readings? He was clearly anxious about attending the surgery; the BP was recorded in the evening; and he had had a long wait prior to being seen. A third BP reading should be taken. I explained that although the readings were high no decision would be useful until we had a series of readings and asked him to return in three days to morning surgery for a repeat check.

The protocol suggested that patients with a reading of 200/120 mmHg should be seen weekly, whereas those with more moderate readings can be reviewed fortnightly or monthly, depending on other risk factors. I advised him not to eat for 4 hours (so he could take fasting lipids) or to have exercised for half an hour prior to his next appointment. I also requested he bring a urine sample for routine analysis.

At the end of his first appointment what risk factors for coronary heart disease should have been identified? Male sex; advancing age; family history; and stress.

The second appointment had been made in the heart disease prevention clinic where 20-minute appointments allow enough time for a detailed assessment. The aim of the clinic is to:

- assess lifestyle and identify a number of risk factors for coronary heart disease

- educate about risk factors and their link to coronary heart disease

- provide support to those who wish to reduce risk by making lifestyle changes

- identify appropriate treatment regimes where necessary

- educate those who require medication about all aspects of their drugs.

Patients who attend the clinic are likely to do so over a long period of time. The nurse aims to begin to build a trusting relationship with them and their families by adopting a non-judgemental approach.

James' assessment found that he was a non-smoker with a strong family history of ischaemic heart disease. His pulse was recorded at 88 beats per minute and regular. He was a teetotaller, enjoyed his food and his body mass index was 28 – making him a little over weight (body mass is weight in kg/height in m; normal range 20–25 for men and 18.3–23.6 for women). He felt that his diet was fairly low in fat, but admitted to liberally adding salt to his food. He took no exercise apart from very occasional gardening and drove everywhere. He admitted to feeling quite stressed most of the time.

Urinalysis was tested for glucose to exclude diabetes and protein to eliminate renal disease. Bloods were taken to establish baseline readings of urea and electrolytes, liver function and fasting lipids, fasting blood sugar, uric acid and a full blood count. (Ten per cent of all patients with elevated blood pressure will have a diagnosable and treatable cause, that is secondary hypertension caused by, for example, renal disease and these conditions must be screened for.) Blood pressure was recorded on three occasions at five minute intervals and the lowest reading 172/98 mmHg was recorded.

As it now appeared likely that James was going to have a degree of hypertension I gave him some literature produced by the stroke association, about the causes and effects of high blood pressure, to take home. When giving patient information leaflets it is important to be sure of their content, be aware of who has produced them and whether there is any bias in the way the information is presented. Also consider whether the information and evidence presented is up to date and accurate. Above all, assess whether the patient benefit from the leaflet, remembering that we all have different lifestyles and that some patients cannot read?

I arranged a third appointment in two weeks time for both a final blood pressure check and an electrocardiogram to identify any evidence of left ventricular hypertrophy. I also asked him to invite his wife to come with him to the next appointment. Involvement of his partner may aid his understanding of the need for change, provide support and improve compliance to any proposed lifestyle changes. I suggested that it might be useful if he kept a food diary for the week prior to his next appointment. Before you can suggest any constructive advice you need to assess the patients' current intake and to establish why they prefer certain foods. A food diary gives an overall idea of the types of food eaten, helps to establish meal pattern and some lifestyle factors, such as the number of takeaways.

Maintaining a food diary is time consuming and if the patient is not motivated they may present an inaccurate record (Gilbert, 1997). The food diary revealed that, when compared to the national food guide for healthy eating (Health Education Authority, 1994), an average day would comprise between one and two portions of fruit and vegetables, seven portions of bread, cereal and potatoes, four portions of dairy foods, three portions of fatty and sugary foods, and between three and four portions of meat, fish and alternatives. In addition salt was added to food although none was used in the cooking.

Blood test results showed that uric acid was slightly raised; fasting lipids showed cholesterol 8.5 mmol/l, triglycerides 1.9 mmol/l, while other results were normal. The electrocardiogram did show mild left ventricular hypertrophy; final blood pressure was 170/98 mmHg. The protocol based on the British Hypertension Societies management guidelines identifies optimal blood pressure treatment targets are systolic blood pressure <140 mmHg and diastolic blood pressure <85 mmHg; the minimum acceptable level of control (audit standard) recommended is <150/<90 mmHg. A further assessment of James' risk of coronary heart disease could be made using the cardiac risk assessor identified by the British Hypertension Society (1999) – ideally he should have a 10-year CHD risk ⩽15 per cent. Therefore, James demonstrated multiple risk factors and was significantly hypertensive.

What lifestyle changes would James benefit from making?

- *Dietary*: increase fibre and, decrease total fat intake, particularly saturated fat; use a salt replacement
- *Activity*: gradually build up to 20-minutes gentle daily exercise.

The focus of the third appointment is patient education. The nurse moves into a supportive/educative role. She has a responsibility to explain the relevant facts so that the client can decide whether they wish to alter their lifestyle to reduce their level of risk of coronary heart disease. This involves explaining what blood pressure is and the affect it can have on the body. Once that is understood you can then explain how changes in lifestyle may improve the blood pressure. At this point some patients may also want to know what the treatment options are if lifestyle change is not sufficiently effective. James, however, made it clear he did not want to discuss treatment and emphasised that he did not want to 'start tablets'.

James had read the literature and so I got him to tell me what he understood high blood pressure to be. He asked me whether rising blood pressure was part of the ageing process. I explained that although blood pressure appears to rise with age, the research indicates that it is not due to age but rises in response to lifestyle. I then began to explain how lifestyle change could improve his blood pressure significantly. In mild hypertensives, this reduction can be up to 10.6/8.1 mmHg. (The treatment of mild hypertension research group, 1991).

I explained that the risk of developing CHD rises progressively with increase in serum cholesterol but that conversely a reduction of 0.6 mmols in dietary cholesterol is estimated to lower the risk of CHD by up to 80 per cent in a 70-year-old (Law, 1994). I explained that this sort of reduction could be achieved by moderate dietary changes such as increasing fibre, eating oily fish weekly, increasing intake of fruit and vegetables to a minimum of five portions per day and cutting out pastries and cheese. I also noted that clients who follow a low fat diet almost always lose weight and this would also help reduce his blood pressure; loss of 5 kg in weight has been shown to correlate with a reduction in blood pressure of 5 mmHg (Sever *et al.*, 1993).

We discussed salt reduction and how research had shown that by decreasing your salt intake by 3 gms per day (0.5 teaspoonful) blood pressure could be reduced by 5 mmHg (Lakin *et al.*, 1996). We talked about how an inactive, sedentary lifestyle increases the risk of CHD and stroke (Lee Tai *et al.*, 1997). I explained that regular physical activity can help to keep weight down and heart rate and blood pressure responses to a lower level, but that exercise should be gradually increased. We briefly discussed stress. I explained that there was no clear evidence to show high blood pressure is caused by stress, but that from my experience with other clients there was often benefit derived from looking at ways to reduce stress such as relaxation exercises.

After some discussion, James and his wife decided that the initial effort should be focused on his diet and that this would be given a three-month trial. How would the suggested dietary changes reduce cholesterol? Adding more fruit and vegetables would increase the antioxidants that are important in the prevention of heart disease because they prevent free radical damage to circulating low-density lipo-protein cholesterol (Morrell and Lynas, 1998). Increasing soluble fibre lowers cholesterol (Gilbert,

1997) and increasing the consumption of oily fish, for example, mackerel or herring twice a week may increase HDL cholesterol concentration and have a protective effect against CHD (Effective Health Care, 1998). Any nurse working with a patient who is trying to make fundamental lifestyle changes will need to be aware of, and able to apply, the most appropriate model of health behaviour. Prochaska and Diclemente (1986) argue that an understanding of the process of change is the key to being an effective support to the client. This client centred model adopts a very positive approach in that it recognises that human relapse is a natural part of behavioural change.

When James arrived for his third appointment, having read the literature, he was at the contemplative stage. He was aware that his weight might be affecting his blood pressure and that his diet could be improved. He wanted to know what evidence there was that his diet was linked to blood pressure and increased risk of CHD. By the end of the appointment, he had already reached the phase where he was preparing to make the change and recognised that the benefits of making the change appeared too many to ignore. The nurses' role now is to help the client prepare to make the change and to explore alternative strategies. Through discussion it emerged that Mr Smith had never liked fruit or vegetables since being made to eat cabbage as a child; that the family had a routine of having a supper of cheese, butter and biscuits at 9 pm each evening; and that Mr Smith felt that his food would be tasteless without salt. I explained about salt replacement and asked him to consider ways he could incorporate more fibre and suggested fruit juice as an alternative to fruit and vegetables. I asked him to set himself two goals that we could review in a week. He decided on cutting out salt and trying fruit juice.

By the next appointment he was making the changes. His blood pressure was not measured, as the focus of the appointment was to review progress with lifestyle change. Salt had been replaced with a potassium supplement and this was acceptable. He was enjoying three glasses of fruit juice daily and had even tried some of the more unusual vegetables; his wife had made a vegetable soup that he had also enjoyed. In addition they had also changed the supper, replacing the butter and cheese with low fat cream cheese with garlic. Mr Smith felt that this had been a struggle and said he almost 'felt cheated'. I suggested he included something in the supper that was a real treat and he was surprised when I did not veto his wife's suggestion of a finger of chocolate wafer. This emphasises the importance of making sure that the goals set are realistic and achievable.

I met with James twice more in the next month while he maintained the change. Frequent follow-up is important to boost motivation, explore any difficulties and emphasize the benefits of the change (Prochaska and Diclemente, 1986). He had already noticed that his trousers were loose and that he felt less tired. They had adjusted their meal pattern so that supper was now at 6 pm that gave them time to also fit in an evening walk. He had had one relapse when friends had popped around and they had found some Stilton still in the fridge. This emphasizes the importance of preparing clients to change by telling others and clearing food out of the house that you do not want to eat. He had however not eaten as much as usual because he had found the cheese seemed to taste fatty! His blood pressure was taken and the lowest of three readings showed that it had fallen slightly to 167/95. He had also lost 1.2 kg, which was encouraging. It is important to encourage the patient to take an interest in their hypertension management (REACH, 1998). This involves sharing the blood pressure readings with the patient and identifying a target. I told James that the minimum we should accept was 140/85 mmHg but that ideally it would be better even lower.

Wherever possible lifestyle change should be seen as the first treatment and given a minimum three-month trial period. If the client remains hypertensive treatment is required. Whether or not the cholesterol is treated will depend in part on the number of risk factors as well as the actual cholesterol reading. At three months James' BMI had fallen to 26.6 and his cholesterol had dropped, but remained high at 7.1. Prior to recording his blood pressure I was careful to ascertain whether he had maintained the lifestyle changes and how he was feeling. He was feeling fitter, had more energy and was enjoying his healthy eating programme. He re-emphasized that he did not want to start treatment. His blood pressure was 165/95 and it seemed it would not reach acceptable levels without treatment.

I asked him what about treatment concerned him and he explained that it was the life long aspect and the possible side effects. I suggested that I gave him some information about the different options for treatment and that he could then decide what he wanted to do. After some discussion we negotiated that he would consider the treatment options, but that he also planned to increase his exercise further and that if while on treatment his blood pressure should fall to below 140/80 mmHg we would consider a further trial without treatment. The British Hypertension Society advises that patient with stable blood pressure and no evidence of end organ damage can have their treatment reduced and occasionally withdrawn, provided lifestyle changes are adhered to and blood pressure is regularly monitored.

The options for treatment are, as identified in the practice protocol, were thiazide diuretics, β-blockers, α-blockers, calcium channel blockers and ace inhibitors. Involving James in the choice of any possible treatment was crucial to compliance. We looked at each group of drugs and how they worked to control BP, the key advantages and side effects (see Table 11.1).

Table 11.1 Patient information about drugs used to treat hypertension

	Mild Diuretic	β-blocker	Ace inhibitor	α-blocker
Drug Names	e.g. Bendrofluazide	e.g. Atenolol	e.g. Lisinopril 2.5 mg–20 mg Captopril 12.5 mg–50 mg Elanapril 5 mg–20 mg	e.g. Cardura
Usual dosage	2.5 mg–5 mg once daily, time to suit you	25–50 mg daily	Lisinopril 1 daily Captopril 3 daily Elanapril 2 daily	1–4 mg daily
Main side effects	These are rare. Increase in number of times and amount of urine passed, rash, occasional impotence, very rarely gout,	Fatigue Dizziness Cold extremities	Cough Occasionally dizziness on sitting or standing, kidney problems Diarrhoea in the elderly Rarely problems with eyes	Dizziness particularly on standing Headaches Palpitations
How they work	Act on kidneys causing an increase in the excretion of and salt in the urine that reduces the circulatory load.	They reduce the effect of adrenaline on the heart that lowers the blood pressure and keeps the heart rate slow and steady.	Angiotensins are hormones produced in the body that regulate blood pressure. By blocking production of angiotensin II this drug causes dilation as well by improving circulation to the kidneys.	Block the effect of receptors in the blood vessels which would normally cause the arterial and venous system to constrict, thus raising blood pressure.
Missed tablet	Don't worry; tablet is mild, take 1 later double dose next day.	Take missed tablet when you remember, don't double the dose.	Take missed tablet later. Do not double the next day's dose	
Self monitoring			We will need to take blood samples to check on your renal function.	

McInnes (1997) suggests that when considering which drug to choose to treat hypertension there are six factors to consider.

- Efficacy in reducing BP
- Tolerability
- Safety
- Compatibility with other drugs
- Modification of outcome

He argues that if all the above are equal consideration should then be given to cost. Acceptability to the patient must also be considered.

Diuretics are recommended by the BHS as a first line antihypertensive agent and they are very cheap. However, two known side effects are an elevation of the levels of plasma cholesterol and uric acid. James' uric acid was already slightly raised and his cholesterol higher than desirable and so I counselled him against this option. He had clearly done his own research as he explained that he would not have considered thiazides because of the potential side effect of impotence. Equally, he had ruled out β-blockers because he was concerned that they might make him more lethargic. I was also aware that β-blockers could have adversely affected plasma lipid levels, although they might have been useful to dampen James' anxiety levels.

We then considered ace inhibitors. These are expensive but generally well tolerated by patients, effective and particularly useful in patients with mild left ventricular dysfunction. James' however, had had a friend who had experienced the side effect of the chronic dry cough, and was not very keen. He was unaware of α-blockers. I explained that this was a drug with a low side effect profile that could be given once daily and that there was some research that suggested that they might have a positive effect on blood cholesterol. (McInnes 1997 notes that a 5 per cent reduction in total cholesterol and LDL, and a similar increase in HDL, have been seen in long term therapy.) It is a treatment that is started with a very low dose and gradually increased as needed. Reluctantly he agreed to consider an α-blocker and I then explained how it worked.

How would you explain the action of an α-blocker to a patient? α-blockers block the action of receptors in the circulation that would normally cause the blood vessels to constrict. We discussed the side effects, the main one being the risk of postural hypotension. This was minimised by Mr Smith agreeing to take the first dose before he went to bed and using a low starting dose of 1 mg daily. I then confirmed my plan of action, carefully explaining my rationale, with the doctor who then prescribed cardura to James. A month later there was clear progress. Mr Smith felt more energetic, weight loss was 0.8 kg and his BP was 155/82 mmHg (lowest of three readings). He had experienced no side effects from the medication. We had agreed a target blood pressure of 140/90 mmHg and after consultation with the doctor increased the dose to 2 mg cardura daily. Eight weeks later his weight was stable and he was eating healthily. His cholesterol was 6.2 mmols/l BP 142/84 mmHg and we agreed that this was acceptable. James is now reviewed on a six monthly basis and his BP is stable.

When evaluating James' care what factors would you consider?

- BP
- Weight loss
- Cholesterol
- Medication compliance
- Patients' views

Attempt was made throughout James' care to involve him in the decisionmaking process and there was a clear rationale behind each decision taken. He felt that he had a clear understanding of the problem and the treatment. All decisions about care were made based on the evidence currently available.

Conclusion

Attempts were made throughout James, care to involve him in the decision making process and there was a clear rationale behind each decision taken. He felt that he had a clear understanding of the problem and the treatment. All decisions about care were made based on the evidence currently available. The government is now focusing General Practice far more on the need for improvement in the management of patients with hypertension through the National Service Framework for Coronary Heart Disease (1997). It is almost inevitable that this will result in practice nurses becoming increasingly involved with this client group. This discussion has attempted to show that with the judicious use of a protocol, support from General Practitioners and appropriate training, the practice nurse can effectively work with patients to help them control their hypertension.

Part V

Setting Up the Nurse Led Clinic

12

The Nurse Led Clinic: Organisation and Responsibility

JAN DAVIS

Health professionals are keen to offer the best care possible to patients and all of us can think of areas that will improve our care to patients. It might be because of a recently read article that highlights an unmet need and stimulates concern, or it could be a particular interest of the health professional. Making decisions about changing care needs careful thought and planning.

In current policy changes aiming to modernise the NHS, the objective is to ensure prompt access to equitable, high quality care wherever a patient is treated (see Box 12.1). There are many influences on and within the healthcare system (see Figure 12.1) that must be taken into account when deciding which services to offer patients. Health centres and surgeries are generally the first point of contact for most people and the government recognized that community nurses and GPs were best placed to understand the health needs of the local population (Department of Health, 1997).

Box 12.1 **The new NHS**

The New NHS will have quality at its heart. Without it, there is unfairness. Every patient who is treated in the NHS wants to know that they can rely on receiving high quality care when they need it. Every part of the NHS, and every one who works in it, should take responsibility for working to improve quality.

Source: Department of Health, *The New NHS, Modern, Dependable* para. 3.2 (1997) Cm 3807: December.

Figure 12.1 Influences on and within the health care system

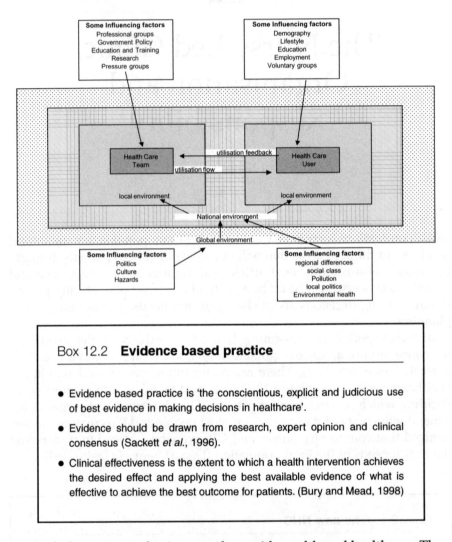

Box 12.2 **Evidence based practice**

- Evidence based practice is 'the conscientious, explicit and judicious use of best evidence in making decisions in healthcare'.

- Evidence should be drawn from research, expert opinion and clinical consensus (Sackett *et al.*, 1996).

- Clinical effectiveness is the extent to which a health intervention achieves the desired effect and applying the best available evidence of what is effective to achieve the best outcome for patients. (Bury and Mead, 1998)

Much discussion today is centred on evidenced-based healthcare. There is a vast pool of information out there, which can be both overwhelming and confusing. It can be very time consuming to search out and read relevant literature. However, with the formation of the National Institute of Clinical Effectiveness and National Service frameworks, guidance will become available on best practice and its implementation, which will be both clinically and cost effective. Information will be released over time. At present, these bodies have only just been formed and become operational and, therefore, the amount of help and guidance will be limited.

Box 12.3 **Key points**

- Guidelines should be based on best practice or if available evidence based practice.
- Offering a structured approach to care will ensure that all patients receive the same care which is of a consistently high standard

---

Primary Care Groups/Trusts will be able to offer help, advice and guidance on implementing new changes in care provision. Each board will have a clinical governance lead, whose remit is to look at improving standards of care and who will be very interested in quality practice initiatives. Primary Care Boards are also being guided by government directives, which aim to promote one or two national strategies for health, for example, coronary heart disease and mental health. They will also be responsible for commissioning services for their local community to best suit local circumstances and need. Linking in with either a national or local strategy will be advantageous, as a lot of advice and help will be available.

However, we should remember that national and local strategies are there to help guide and inform practice, but should not stifle innovation. If, as a health professional you identify a need for which a change in provision of care would bring measurable benefits to patients, then go ahead. Good preparation and planning however, is paramount to ensure its success (see Box 12.2). Work in general practice is rapidly expanding and it makes sense to ensure that the area of practice identified will significantly improve care provision. It is not realistically feasible to change practice in all the areas we would like to and so setting priorities will mean you can tackle topics that obtain the most advantageous results for your efforts (see Box 12.3). Make sure when you research the topic that it is clinically worthwhile and will offer patients an improved service with better outcomes of care. If it offers you the added benefit of professional development, in an area you are interested in then so much the better.

Before you start, consider the resource implications. Do you have the time and commitment to follow the project through? Are there financial implications? Is there someone else in the primary care team who could help you and support your idea? In principal, there must be sufficient support from your colleagues in order for the changes to be made. Box 12.4 outlines steps to take in preparation for improving the care and developing a new service.

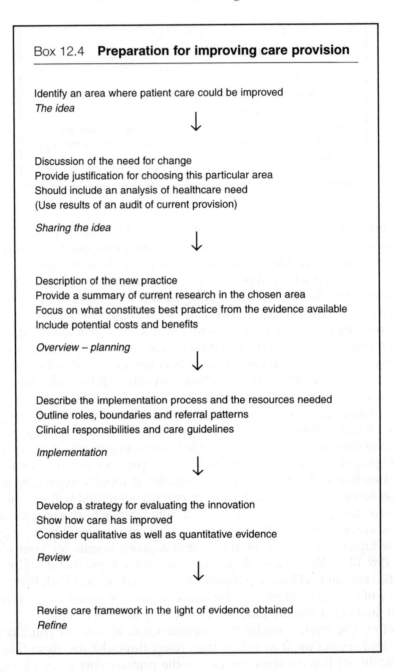

Box 12.4 **Preparation for improving care provision**

Identify an area where patient care could be improved
The idea

Discussion of the need for change
Provide justification for choosing this particular area
Should include an analysis of healthcare need
(Use results of an audit of current provision)

Sharing the idea

Description of the new practice
Provide a summary of current research in the chosen area
Focus on what constitutes best practice from the evidence available
Include potential costs and benefits

Overview – planning

Describe the implementation process and the resources needed
Outline roles, boundaries and referral patterns
Clinical responsibilities and care guidelines

Implementation

Develop a strategy for evaluating the innovation
Show how care has improved
Consider qualitative as well as quantitative evidence

Review

Revise care framework in the light of evidence obtained
Refine

Improving Practice: Developing Clinical Care Guidelines

In developing any clinical care guidelines, a good knowledge base is necessary and provides a secure foundation from which to practice. Decisions need to be made depending on professional background and experience, to develop a framework detailing the area and extent of responsibility and autonomy. This can, and should be, reviewed periodically to enable the nurse to take on additional responsibility as she becomes more experienced. Going through this process will identify training needs.

Developing a clinical care framework to produce guidelines for practice is a valuable process during which the nurse and GP can discuss and negotiate areas of skill and competence and determine levels for referral. When negotiating boundaries for clinical practice the nurse is referred to the UKCC Guidelines for professional practice (UKCC, 1992a). If there are clear role boundaries then there is less opportunity for role conflict. Few professionals are clear about the scope of practice, expertise and competencies, of other disciplines (Paley, 1995). In the past, there has been an emphasis on medicalising care but the thrust forward recently is in recognizing the value of multidisciplinary care so that the patient receives a more holistic approach. Building professional partnerships and the recognition of each other's specific area of expertise and skill enables truly collaborative practice.

Patients should receive quality care and clinical guidelines when developed and used properly can ensure that patients consistently receive high standards of care (see Box 12.5).

Protocols or Guidelines

The terminology is confusing to many as people use these terms interchangeably; it is important to have a clearer understanding of what is meant by them. As the National Institute for Clinical Excellence has been given the brief to lead on the development of national guidelines and standards, the following definitions will undoubtedly be refined. The most widely quoted definition for guidelines to date describes them as:

> Systematically developed statements to assist practitioner decisions about appropriate healthcare for specific clinical circumstances. (Institute of Medicine, 1992)

National guidelines reflect broad statements of good practice and are intended to be adapted for local use (NHSE, 1996). Local clinical guidelines are more specific and can be likened to protocols in that they contain more operational detail (Duff *et al.*, 1996).

Box 12.5 **Organisation of care**

Practice nurse

Compile a register of patients

Devise letter of invitation

Collect patient information leaflets

Attend relevant study days,*
 visit hospital clinics

Organise in-house, multi-disciplinary
 training to expand existing knowledge
 and awareness of new clinic services

Decide on method of recording patient
 care and advice given. Develop or obtain
 record card

Practice manager/practice staff

Organise clinic times, appointments
 and rooms

Advertise new service in practice leaflet,
 put posters/notices up

Send out letters of invitation

Develop recall system for appointments
 and for non-attenders

*General Practitioner/
Practice Nurse*

Decide on aims of initial
 consultation

Plan contents of
 follow-up sessions

Regularly review progress of
 clinic
Referral criteria

Decide on role boundaries,
 so everyone is clear
 on who does what

Liaise with other team mem
 bers involved; immediate
 primary care team, schools
 and school health services,
 social services and voluntary
 organisations, self help
 groups and secondary care
 specialists on referral criteria

Note: *Contact the National Society for Epilepsy for details of courses.

Protocols are documents of clinical recommendations. Although they are more prescriptive, they should allow for clinical judgement. Jenkins (1991) defines protocols as,

Precise guidelines with a structured and logical approach to a closely specified, clinical problem.

More specifically, the main purposes of protocols are identified by Dukes and Stewart (1993) as:

- to assist in diagnosis by providing written recommendations that enable healthcare workers to systematically evaluate health problems
- to improve medical care by setting out best practice and ensuring that the care is co-ordinated by the different clinicians involved
- to predict costs involved and so improve budgetary control
- for legal protection, demonstrating the treatment pathway the clinician has followed
- to present legal and ethical issues to be taken into account when a patient refuses treatment.

Although protocols are protective in that they can be used to provide evidence for the care that is given – in the event of a problem – they can also be used as evidence to show that protocols have not been adhered to. It is necessary for clinicians to state any deviation from protocol in their documentation at the time of delivery of care and the reasons why a particular treatment pathway was not followed to support the changes.

Protocols should not be developed in isolation but as part of a multi-disciplinary approach. In this way, expert opinion and clinical consensus can be utilized to provide sound, clinically effective care.

Principles of Running a Nurse Led Clinic

In general practice many new developments in care have been formalized with the introduction of mini clinics which focus on various areas of care: well person, asthma, diabetes and coronary heart disease prevention being probably the most common, with other innovations such as rheumatoid arthritis, teenage health, psoriasis, epilepsy management in some areas.

Help with appropriate patient information leaflets may be available from relevant drug companies or registered charities/organisations. Taking time to read the choice of literature available, so that it will be geared to the client group, is essential. Do you need to have leaflets in various languages? Consideration needs to be given to whether the care is best provided in the form of a clinic at a specified time of the week devoted to solely seeing patients with that particular health need, or whether appointments can be offered within the normal surgery times. Aspects to bear in mind will be the type of clients the new practice will attract for example if it focuses on teenage health issues then offering appointments in school time hours would be pointless.

Letters of invitation, or a mixture of all three approaches outlined above, can recruit patients to clinics by self referral, or referral from other members of the primary care team. It may be that the availability of consulting rooms will influence the decision of when and how the care can be provided. If you require a GP to be on hand, then this could be another factor to take into account. With a bit of ingenuity and forethought most problems can be overcome!

Once the guidelines have been developed the actual structure to providing the new service needs to be put in place. Box 12.5 outlines the steps in preparation for running a nurse led clinic.

Conclusion

Developing guidelines based on research, clinical consensus and expert opinion, to inform and structure practice enables *consistency* of care and improves the *quality* of care given. Link with the primary care group lead on clinical governance for ideas on current trends in improving practice. Ensure that all members of the primary care team are involved right from the start; they might not need to take an active part but it will help if they are supportive of the innovation and keep them informed at all stages. You should consider patient involvement in the evaluation stage and seek feedback once the project is up and running. The process will identify training needs and the resources required. However, good preparation is the key to a successful project.

13

Improving Care for the Patient with Epilepsy

JAN DAVIS

This chapter covers the topic of epilepsy as a project designed to show the type of information needed and some of the steps to be taken to develop improved care of patients in general practice with epilepsy. It outlines some of the background information required to help in understanding the condition. It is not intended to be a definitive text on the subject of epilepsy. Readers are encouraged to obtain further; more detailed information from books, journals, specialists and relevant organisations for more in-depth knowledge. It suggests how general practice can initiate improvement in practice-based care by audit and evaluation of that care. The nurse's role in management and provision of appropriate health information is described using a case study scenario. Utilizing information from Chapter 12, it is intended to provide clear, simple, practical information to enable any health professional in primary care with an interest in epilepsy, to improve the care of patients. (Names of epilepsy organisations and appropriate further reading materials can be found in the Appendix.)

Epilepsy is the most common serious neurological condition affecting up to 500 000 people in the UK (Wallace *et al.*, 1997). Care is often ineffective with poor structure, a lack of follow-up, ineffective use of drugs, poor seizure control and a lack of information for patients and their families. Misdiagnosis is a significant problem. Too often patients with epilepsy are seen in hospital by non-neurologists. There is a dearth of specialist neurologists in the UK with only 21 clinics specifically for epilepsy and seven special centres; one-tenth the number of neurologists provided in the Netherlands, for an equivalent population (Duncan and Hart, 1993).

Epilepsy and the social stigma surrounding the condition has many negative consequences for patients and their families, influencing many aspects of their lives. The word epilepsy still evokes fear and superstition for many people and raises both personal and family anxiety levels. Some patients may have associated learning disabilities. For patients to benefit,

231

general practice management and care from specialist centres needs to be co-ordinated. The Epilepsy Needs document recommends that people with epilepsy should be seen at regular intervals by the primary care team, at least annually (Brown *et al.*, 1993). Nurses can make a valuable contribution to the care of patients with epilepsy in general practice. (Ridsdale *et al.*, 1997).

Nurse run clinics are established in other areas of chronic disease management such as asthma and diabetes and have led to significant improvements in patient care. Providing structured care of epilepsy would lead to an increase in clinical workload and currently there is no remuneration for providing such a service. GPs, however, do receive a fee for providing chronic disease management for patients with diabetes and asthma.

Definition

Epileptic seizures are due to an intermittent and temporary disturbance in the brain, which produces some or all of the following symptoms:

- disturbance of consciousness or awareness;
- alterations of bodily movement, sensation or posture.'

Clinical signs and symptoms may take many different forms depending on which area of the brain's cortex is affected. Epilepsy has, therefore, many causes and presentations. Seizures can be seen as symptoms of an underlying brain dysfunction, but often no obvious causes are found.

Many people have a single seizure episode at some time in their lives but a diagnosis of epilepsy is seldom made on the basis of this. In Britain the term epilepsy is presently applied to patients who have recurrent (two or more) seizures. Febrile or neonatal seizures are excluded. Most readers will remember being taught about grand mal and petit mal seizures and might have heard about subsequent classifications of tonic–clonic seizures. A newer classification based on whether the seizures are gener-alised in nature, or partial and arising from a focal area in the brain, is becoming more widely used.

It is important to correctly classify the seizures experienced as different types of epilepsy have different causes, management and outlook. The characteristics of seizures depend upon the area of the brain affected. It is important to exclude any underlying causes such as a cerebral tumour, although these are rare. By correctly classifying seizures, optimal treatment can be instituted, especially important in some of the epilepsy syndromes where a cluster of signs, symptoms and findings from investigations, together with the onset age, provide better guidance on the prognosis and treatment choices than seizure type alone. Most epilepsy syndromes occur in childhood and should be managed by specialists.

The prognosis is encouraging but depends on the type of epilepsy and its underlying cause. Studies have shown that over 70 per cent of patients with epilepsy become seizure free (Sander, 1993).

Epidemiology

There are difficulties in establishing precise epidemiological statistics for a condition like epilepsy. Diagnostic accuracy is a common problem as there is a variety of other conditions which may be confused with epilepsy, such as syncope or psychogenic attacks. Diagnosis is retrospective, as it can only be diagnosed by taking a history of the event or by a chance observation of the seizure. It is a clinical diagnosis and depends upon the patient's account of his seizures or more importantly, the quality of description given by an eyewitness. Between seizures the patients clinical examination and investigations may be perfectly normal.

Classification of Seizures

Partial Seizures (seizures begin locally, most commonly from temporal lobe)

Simple partial: uncommon, and not always indicating the presence of an underlying abnormality such as an intracerebral lesion. Clinical presentation depends on cortical area in which electrical discharge occurs.

Temporal lobe seizures may result in the patient experiencing powerful smells, tastes or *deja-vu*.

Frontal lobe seizures may result in jerking of one limb 'Jacksonian seizure' or eyes and head turning to one side.

Parietal lobe seizures (less common) may result in tingling sensations or jerking down one side of the body.

Occipital seizures (less common) may cause flashing lights.

Generally sudden onset, but brief episodes. No impairment of consciousness

Complex partial: consciousness impaired at some point in the seizure; patient awareness affected. Automatisms are a common feature of these types of seizures, examples are smacking of lips, fidgeting with clothing, wandering aimlessly.

Partial seizures secondarily generalized.

Both simple and complex seizures can spread to become generalised seizures.

Generalised Seizures

Tonic–clonic: commonest generalised seizure type. Person falls to the ground, becomes rigid with rapid onset of cyanosis. There may be incontinence of urine or faeces or biting of tongue followed by rhythmical jerking of limbs. May last for a few minutes after which person enters post ictal phase. May complain of headache and be confused, feel tired and want to sleep.

Absence: also known as 'Petit- mal'. Usual onset in childhood and adolescence. Blank staring, fluttering of eyelids and nodding of head may occur.

Myoclonic: abrupt very brief, involuntary jerking movements. Often occur shortly after waking or before going to bed. Recovery is immediate.

Atonic: Sudden loss of tone in postural muscles, patient falls. Sometimes referred to as 'drop attacks'. Injuries may occur.

Tonic: Sudden increase in muscle tone in body, patient becomes rigid and usually falls to ground. No jerking, injuries may occur.

Unclassified seizures: (inadequate or incomplete data to make it sufficiently possible to classify).

Morag – Case Study 1

As a young girl, Morag was diagnosed as having migraine and was well controlled on simple analgesic medication. As she became older, she tried various alternative treatments such as acupuncture and homeopathic remedies. She was not overly troubled by these episodes and found that the alternative treatments helped considerably. In her mid twenties, Morag found it increasingly difficult to control her headaches with either simple analgesia or with alternative medicine. She saw her GP with her boyfriend with whom she now shared a home. On close questioning and going back over her history some doubt was cast on the diagnosis of migraine. When asked if the headaches affected her when sleeping, her boyfriend described being woken by loud noises as if Morag was smacking her lips together during the night prior to when Morag had complained of a headache. He would try to rouse her but Morag would have no recollection of it in the morning. They had laughed about it before without realizing its significance. The GP discussed the possibility of epilepsy, referring Morag to a neurologist. Being aware of the diagnosis she began to recognise minor episodes where she would inexplicably find herself not being able to get the right word out or being confused adding simple sums. A diagnosis of temporal lobe epilepsy, with partial complex seizures was made.

Another problem in determining the exact epidemiology of epilepsy is that the patient may be unaware of the seizures and not seek help, or conceal their condition because of the stigma attached to epilepsy. For the epidemiology to be accurate it is important that all cases are included. An active case is defined as a person with epilepsy who has had at least one seizure in the previous five years regardless of treatment. Inactive cases are defined as a person with epilepsy with no seizures for five years or more and receiving treatment (remission with treatment), or a person with epilepsy with no seizures for more than five years and not receiving treatment (remission without treatment) (Sander and Shorvon, 1996).

Prevalence

The number of all new and old cases of a disease, or occurrences of an event at a given time.

Incidence

Incidence describes the number of new cases per given population. The prevalence of active epilepsy is around 4–10 per 1000. This equates to each GP with an average list size of 2000 patients, having between eight and 20 patients registered with active epilepsy. The incidence of epilepsy has been estimated to be up to 100 cases per 100 000 persons. While up to 30 per cent of patients will develop chronic epilepsy, many will cease to have seizures.

Lifetime prevalence rates (the risk of having the condition at some time in one's life) are therefore much higher. It is estimated that between 1.5 and 5 per cent of the population will have one non-febrile seizure episode (Sander and Shorvon, 1996). The incidence is relatively high in the first decade of life, particularly in the first year. Rates fall in early adult life but increase in later life, mainly as a result of seizures due to cerebrovascular disease. Rates are higher in males than females. (Sander and Shorvon, 1987). The mortality rate is raised among people with epilepsy (Cockerell *et al.*, 1994), with a recognised and increased risk of sudden unexplained death, particularly in young men (Leestma *et al.*, 1989).

Aetiology

There are numerous causes of epilepsy including congenital or genetic deformities, birth trauma, head injury, brain tumours, cerebrovascular disease and infections, but in 60 to 70 per cent of cases no cause will be found. However, with more extensive investigation such as brain MRI a more accurate picture of the aetiology of epilepsy may become apparent.

Epileptic seizures can be triggered by a number of recognised precipitants. They can occur in patients with epilepsy as well as in susceptible people without previous seizures. The most common triggers for people with epilepsy are stress and emotional upsets, over tiredness and excessive alcohol. Flickering lights, menstruation and high fevers can also precipitate seizures.

Audit

Initial audit of the care of patients with epilepsy will help to identify strengths and weaknesses in the care provided, providing the impetus to improve services. As the number of patients with epilepsy is not large the work should not be too time consuming. Audits of patient records of the process of care for people with epilepsy have consistently shown that there is great potential for improvement (Buck *et al.*, 1996; Taylor, 1987). The main difficulties in the care of people with epilepsy broadly seem to be:

- lack of systematic follow-up
- inappropriate polypharmacy
- patient non-compliance with medication
- failure of GP–patient communication
- low levels of patient knowledge

(Thapar, 1996)

Some areas in the UK with primary care audit groups are able to provide funding to undertaking an audit. Initially these groups, when formed in 1990, were called MAAG (Medical Audit Advisory Groups) and every health authority had one. The position is less clear today: some groups are now known as EQUIP (Enhancing quality in primary care), or PCAG (Primary Care Audit Groups). Other areas have relatively little funding for audit but it is still worth contacting the local health authority for information or the local Primary Care Group may be able to help.

Ideas on How to Obtain your List of Relevant Patients

To find patients with active epilepsy, search on read code F25, if you use disease codes. This type of search may reveal patient's names whose epilepsy is now inactive. So, combine this search with a computer search on epileptic drugs.

Drug List

- carbamazepine (tegretol, tegretol retard)
- sodium valporate (epilim, epilim chrono)
- phenytoin (epanutin)
- ethosuximide (zarontin, emeside)
- vigabatrin (sabril)
- clobazam (frisium)
- clonazepam (rivotril)
- phenobarbitome (luminal, prominal)
- primidone (mysoline)
- acetazolomide (diamox)
- lamotrigine (lamictal)
- gabapentin (neurontin)
- valproic acid (convulex)

This search list includes patients on drugs for example, carbamazine for non-epilepsy indications such as trigeminal neuralgia and for chronic pain, or prevention of migraine or depression.

Once you have checked your final list of active epileptic patients, try to keep this list accurate and up to date.

Suggested Areas of Information to Collect

- Practice list size
- Number and percentage of patients identified with active epilepsy
- Gender and age of patient
- Number of fits recorded in past year (include fit free)

- Annual review of epilepsy
- Last hospital consultant visit
- Medication–monotherapy/polytherapy
- Compliance with medication (can be checked by looking at prescribing patterns over a period of 3–6 months)
- Contraceptive advice
- Driving advice

Remember the more complicated the audit the more time it takes to collect evidence based practice.

Epilepsy is an individual disorder affecting people *physically* in different ways depending on the type of seizures experienced and how people respond *emotionally* and *socially* to epilepsy. In advising the patient, information on the condition and explanations of the side effects of medications are only two aspects of the management of epilepsy. What the patients want is continued support. Nurses can provide time to support patients by providing the relevant information, for example, for the young adult starting work or learning to drive; for married couples on family planning issues and future pregnancies. Increased communication can help some way towards lessening the feelings of isolation and frustration that people with epilepsy sometimes feel.

There are several documents that nurses interested in improving epilepsy services can read to help formulate their own guidelines and there are courses to attend from one day to several days or distance learning packages to follow. The following list gives sources of information.

- Cumbria Medical Audit Advisory Group (1992) Cumbrian standard for the management of patients with epilepsy. Carlisle: Cumbria Medical audit Advisory Group.
- Doncaster epilepsy working group (1992). Guidelines for epilepsy in Doncaster. Doncaster: Doncaster epilepsy working group.
- Martin, E. (1992) 'Guidelines for the care of patients suffering from epilepsy', in *Epilepsy – a general practice problem*, London: Royal College of General Practitioners.
- R. O'Connor, J. Cox and M. Coughlan (1992) *Guidelines for the diagnosis and management of epilepsy in general practice*, Dublin, Republic of Ireland: Irish College of General Practitioners.
- Wellcome Foundation (1993) *Epilepsy liaison nurse programme: a management protocol for epilepsy in general practice*, Crewe: Wellcome Foundation.

The Evidence of Need

Studies made during the 1990s have increasingly focused on patient perceptions of epilepsy. One found that the main concerns were about the inability to drive, unpredictability of seizures, employment, learning and cognitive difficulties and psychosocial issues (Hayden *et al.*, 1992). Lack of knowledge about epilepsy and pregnancy, with concerns over the effect of medication on the foetus and the safety of breastfeeding were highlighted. Although response rates were low (33.7 per cent) the number of suitable replies sampled was 517. Dawkins *et al.*, (1993) in a study of 61 patients looked at knowledge and attitude among people with and without epilepsy. There was little difference in knowledge about the nature of epilepsy, its aetiology and seizure triggers between the two groups. Similar concerns identified in the previous study were expressed about the unpredictability of seizures and the effects on pregnancy and child-rearing, with worries over the side effects of medication and dependence.

It has been shown that many people with epilepsy experience some degree of psycho-social problems, although only in a few are they considered to be severe problems. Of greatest concern was the fear of seizures and the fear of stigma in employment (Chaplin *et al.*, 1992). The effect of poorly controlled epilepsy increases the isolation and stigmatisation of patients. Men who had seizures within the previous six months had a three-chance of feeling stigmatised, with an increased risk of developing depression (Ridsdale *et al.*, 1996). Those patients who are well controlled, with no seizures, were less likely to feel stigmatised.

Fewer educational qualifications and higher rates of unemployment were found in patients with epilepsy (Elwes *et al.*, 1991) although this was not found to be true in a subsequent study (Dawkins *et al.*, 1993). Although no statistical evidence was found to support reduced employment levels among epilepsy patients, results showed that patients themselves perceived it as affecting their employment chances. This perception should be addressed when supporting families.

Current Levels of Care

Although it is the most common serious neurological condition, there are few specialist epilepsy clinics in the UK and fewer neurologists per head of population than other specialisms, and the overall care of patients with epilepsy has been reported as poor (Brown *et al.*, 1993). Over 90 per cent of patients are referred to hospital from first presentation in general practice but after initial assessment and treatment are discharged back to the care of their GP, who most people think of as the doctor most responsible for their care (Jacoby, 1993). The 'Epilepsy Needs' document recommends that patients should be seen regularly (at least annually) by the primary care health team (Brown *et al.*, 1993).

Studies show that patients are not being counselled on various issues, from side effects of drugs prescribed for epilepsy, possible interactions with other drugs and alcohol, to information about self help groups (Buck *et al.*, 1996; Ridsdale *et al.*, 1996). In a postal survey of over 400 patients with epilepsy, respondents revealed that they would appreciate an increase in the provision of services and information (Chappell, 1992).

Aims of Management

Management should focus on correctly classifying epilepsy at diagnosis, preventing seizures with the least number and dosage of medications, and identifying and addressing possible effects on patients' lifestyles. Counselling and current, accurate advice are important aspects of care.

Nurses providing care for patients with epilepsy should be knowledgeable over a range of areas so that accurate information is provided and any misconceptions are dispelled. An understanding of the condition will enable patients to adjust and manage their epilepsy confidently. Knowledge of common triggers will assist patients in recognising personal precipitating factors and avoid further seizures. Over time, as new problems arise, sharing management with patients by providing continuity of care, will give tremendous support. Good communication skills and an individualised approach are essential. Some patient groups have specific needs.

Groups with specific needs

- Newly diagnosed patients
- Women of childbearing age
- Children
- Adolescents
- People with learning disabilities
- Elderly people

Using the following case history some of the psycho-social and lifestyle issues will be highlighted.

Kim – a Case History

One summer afternoon Kim, a 30-year-old married woman was out shopping with her son Ben aged 5. Her husband was called to the local A&E department after Kim had been taken there, following a witnessed tonic–clonic seizure. Kim was a healthy woman with no previous seizures. Before the seizure she reported coming out of the shopping mall into bright sunshine. The next thing Kim remembered was coming to, in the ambulance. Outside the shop where Kim collapsed, a former nurse witnessing the incident, told the ambulance men that Kim had had a grand mal seizure. She described seeing Kim on the floor with rhythmical shaking of limbs and then a short period of unconsciousness. There was no incontinence. On the journey to the hospital Kim was reported by the ambulance men as being mainly incoherent. After assessment in A&E, immediate tests were normal; she was referred to hospital for a follow up appointment with the neurologist but advised to see her GP meanwhile. Kim felt tired for the rest of the day and complained of a headache.

What Immediate Issues are there for Kim?

Many people on being diagnosed as having a seizure find it difficult to accept. Kim initially refused to accept the diagnosis. She was advised not to drive. She insisted that her husband speak to the woman who witnessed the incident and continued to drive after a few days. Her GP organised some tests including an EEG, which was reported as normal and referred Kim to the nurse run, general practice neurology clinic. The nurse was able to listen to Kim's concerns and help her understand how the diagnosis had been reached. Many conditions can be confused with epilepsy but because the witness was reliable and it was obvious that there had been a period of confusion (post ictal phase) the diagnosis of a generalised seizure was made. Her son had also described his mummy 'as falling down and shaking'.

Kim should be told that around 5 per cent of people experience a seizure at some point in their lives, often without any known cause. As epilepsy is the term given to patients generally having had more than one seizure at present it is not a definite diagnosis. Kim was advised that she would be unable to drive for at least the next year and this was recorded in the notes. Kim worked full time and although there were many difficulties to be overcome with regard to travelling, she recognized the importance of complying with the regulations.

What are the DVLC Regulations with Regard to Seizures?

It is important that following a seizure patients are aware of driving regulations and nurses should discuss the legalities and document in the notes the main aspects covered during the consultation. Laws regarding driving and epilepsy differ from country to country; and information should be sought from the appropriate authorities.

In the UK information can be obtained from the Driving and Vehicle Licensing Authority (DVLA) in Swansea or from the Epilepsy Association. When a person has a single fit and already has a driving licence, that person must notify the DVLA and stop driving until further notice. If no evidence of epilepsy is shown on clinical examination and after full investigations with the applicant being free from further seizures for a period of one year, then reapplication can be made to the DVLA. Medical information will be requested from the applicant's doctor. When a person with epilepsy wishes to apply for a driving licence for the first time, the normal application form should be filled out and sent to the DVLA, who will request further information from the applicant about the epilepsy and information will be requested from their doctor once the patients consent has been obtained.

Licences are generally issued for one to three years provided all the normal requirements have been fulfilled and the applicant has been free of seizures for one year with or without treatment.

First Aid for Seizures

What advice can you give to Kim's husband in the event of another seizure?

Witnessing seizures can be quite frightening, but it is important to remember a few simple actions to help minimise injury. During the attack the main aim should be to protect the person from injury. *Only* if they are in a dangerous place such as the top of stairs is it necessary to move them, otherwise putting something soft under their head and neck to give support is appropriate. No one should try to restrict limbs or put anything into their mouths during a seizure. Once the seizure has subsided then the patient should be turned on their side to assist recovery and breathing observed. Any excess mucous should be wiped away. Anyone witnessing a seizure should time it. Generally, medical help is not required provided the patient regains consciousness within 10 minutes. If the seizure lasts longer or further seizures occur then medical help should be summoned.

Other Information

Kim reports another seizure. The consultant starts Kim on an anti epileptic drug (AED). What information will Kim need to have?

- The purpose of the medication
- Importance of compliance with medication
- Knowledge of side effects
- What to do if a dose is missed, vomiting occurs, or a trip abroad is planned
- Use of over the counter preparations and interactions with AEDs
- Use of contraceptive pill. The importance of pre-conceptual counselling. Advice must be sought *pre-conceptually* about medication and pregnancy as some drugs can affect the fetus
- Alcohol and AEDs
- Free prescriptions.

Safety Issues

- Avoid open fires or fit secure fireguards
- Fit safety glass in windows and doors. Replace any glass coffee tables
- Use a low level bed
- Keep bathroom door unlocked or fit a lock that can be opened in an emergency from the outside
- Encourage showers instead of baths
- Swimming is possible but only in the presence of someone who is aware of the condition and has life saving skills
- Smokers should avoid smoking alone indoors.

Anyone newly diagnosed with epilepsy will need time to express their feelings. Patients have many initial concerns and can be frightened about what the future holds. The nurse is able to provide time to answer Kim's questions and to judge the right time to introduce new information. Encouraging Kim to join local self help groups or an Epilepsy Association will provide a further source of support and information.

Conclusion

Epilepsy is a complex disorder. Despite being the most common serious neurological condition it is a poorly understood condition surrounded by prejudice and stigma. Misdiagnosis is a serious problem; diagnostic accuracy is improved if there is a good eye witness account. There are numerous causes of epilepsy but in many cases no obvious cause will be found. For many patients the prognosis for remission is good.

Auditing the current level of provision of epilepsy care in general practice will highlight areas to focus on to improve the level of service and enable a structured approach to its provision. There is evidence to support patient's belief that they are not given enough information about their condition and management of medication. Current provision of services is inadequate and improving practice based care can make a valuable contribution to the overall delivery of quality care. Using nursing skills to provide a personalised approach can help alleviate anxiety felt by patients. Listening to patients' concerns and a knowledgeable nurse able to address worries can do much to provide the confidence patients need to manage the condition and look to the future positively.

Part VI

Professional
Issues

14

Clinical Effectiveness

SHIRLEY CROUCH

This book has considered the knowledge, skills, and attitudes required by the nurse in order to be proactive with patients who have chronic disease. The responsibilities and role of the nurse in primary care have been emphasized, particularly as this specific role is now accepted as a discreet area of specialist practice. Practice nursing is identified as one of the eight specialist categories within the discipline of community healthcare nursing. (UKCC, 1994). The nurse in the primary care setting has the same responsibilities as any nurse in any care environment, but as the scope of primary care nursing is developing and diversifying, some specific issues related to primary care nursing need to be considered in more detail.

This chapter will outline the professional issues related to this specialist role. Particular emphasis will be given to the issue of accountability in relation to acquiring enhanced skills as nurse prescribing becomes acknowledged as part of the nurses' role in primary care; nurses within this specialist area might find themselves targeted by pharmaceutical companies, necessitating a consideration of the ethics of product endorsement.

Professional Accountability

The nurse can take guidance from three main documents for their professional accountability. These are the Code of Practice Conduct, (UKCC, 1992a), the Scope of Professional Practice, (UKCC, 1992c) and the Guidelines for Professional Practice, (UKCC, 1996). These are issued by the United Kingdom Central Council for Nursing, Midwifery and Health Visiting and are based on ethico-legal principles. They are there to enable the nurse to use them in her work in order to care, honour and protect the client, but also to act as a vehicle for the nurse to make professional decisions regarding client care; acknowledge professional responsibilities to colleagues and be aware of his/her own professional responsibilities to self and to society as a whole. As the UKCC is charged through

Act of Parliament (The Nurse, Midwives and Health Visitors Act, 1974 – the Nursing and Midwifery Council from 2001) with maintaining standards of the profession, the code of conduct is a binding document, which must be adhered to. Transgression can constitute professional misconduct.

However, these documents are not intended as a set of rules, but to provide a framework for nurses in practice to develop their professional nursing skills and knowledge in order to best meet the needs of their patients and clients. Nurses should remember that there is no such thing as vicarious professional liability. The Code of Conduct, Guidelines for Professional Practice and the Scope of Practice make it clear that it is the individual nurse, regardless of the employment situation or geographical location, who is responsible for his or her actions. It is for the individual nurse to determine the scope of practice, the limits of the work which she can take on and to be sure that they are actually competent to take on that work.

As a registered nurse, midwife or health visitor shall act, at all times, in such a manner as to:

- safeguard the interests and well-being of patients and clients

- ensure that no action or omission on your part, or within your sphere of responsibility is detrimental to the interests, conditions or safety of patients and clients

- maintain and improve your professional knowledge and competence

- acknowledge any limitations in your knowledge and competence and decline any duties or responsibilities unless able to perform them in a safe and skilled manner (UKCC, 1992).

It can be seen from these statements within the Code of Conduct that if a nurse feels at any time that she is being asked to undertake activities for which she has not been properly prepared, then she must refrain from carrying out such activities. As the role of the nurse in primary care evolves, it is a necessity that the nurse must be familiar with the contents of these documents and to use these documents to ensure the best possible care is given to their patients.

The White Paper *Choice and Opportunity* (Department of Health, 1996) proposes changing legislation to help nurses and other health professionals develop their contribution to primary care. The Paper also proposes a range of more flexible contract options for practice nurses. Recommendations would facilitate expansion of traditional secondary care services to the primary care sector. Its acceptance will ultimately affect the role and responsibility of the primary care nurse. The scope of practice will provide the means for nursing to develop out of all recognition and if through this motorway of change, responsibilities regarding knowledge skills and competence are acquired, clients will receive a high standard of care from professionals truly accountable for their care, and the progress of nursing. The principles of accountability are the same for all working within the healthcare service. The parameters of accountability will differ from job to job and are determined by an individual's knowledge, competencies and experience, by her sphere of responsibility and by the degree of authority assigned.

Knowledge can be acquired through different routes. Formal education, providing a structured system where levels of knowledge can be measured against preset criteria such as assessments. These formal systems go some way in allowing others within or outwith the profession to identify the individuals' breadth and depth of cognition. Knowledge can be gained informally through interest of a particular sphere of practice or subject area. This knowledge can support formally gained knowledge, but on its own is unreliable, as it is reliant on an individual's motivation and questioning attitude and as it is not tested in any formal way, knowledge may vary from individual to individual. Therefore, it can be seen that the onus of responsibility is clearly incumbent upon the individual to exercise critical judgement of one's own professional knowledge.

Competencies refer to the levels of skills exercised in performing a role. All nurses have predetermined competencies that must be formally assessed and achieved. (Rule 18, Statutory Instrument 1983 No. 8673). Recipients of care, as well as colleagues, have a right to expect expertise in line with the nurses' qualifications. Competencies are not static and, like knowledge, are developed both formally and informally. The nurse in practice who seeks to enhance her/his role requires competencies. Clinical audit and clinical supervision are two methods of developing and measuring competence and are being developed more widely in various spheres of healthcare practice (Lowry, 1998).

Experience is gained by practising skills, questioning one's own and others' practice, and by searching for and incorporating new knowledge. As evidence based practice and risk assessment become every day practices, 'experience' will be acknowledged as a key component of accountability and it's value recognized when considering the progress of a practitioner from novice to expert. Responsibility is the obligation to perform certain functions on behalf of an organisation, when considering a role; the nurse should scrutinise the job descriptions and will on appointment sign a contract accepting the responsibilities of the post. Qualifications reflect the responsibilities of the role and as the post becomes more specialised and developmental, so the scope of responsibilities widen.

A newly qualified nurse in practice would expect a discreet area of responsibility focused primarily on direct patient care. As knowledge and experience increase, the boundaries of responsibility will shift and the focus may change to specialist practice requiring expert knowledge and skills, such as standard setting, auditing, leadership, innovation, mentorship and self development. It is the responsibility of the individual to know the limitations of his/her knowledge, competencies and experience and to practice within them, but there is also a responsibility on other professionals, particularly nurses who are directed by the code of conduct to know the boundaries of practice and to ensure that practitioners are not coerced or induced to expand beyond their present limits.

Authority has several contexts; it can refer to a position within an organisation with limits and controls. Authority can be granted and can be delegated. Authority is not power; power is only a part of authority. Authority is also linked with boundaries set by knowledge and competence and one will be held accountable if these are breached. It is in the delegation of authority that power is sometimes abused. There are still occasions in practice when nurses are asked, by a superior, to act in a more senior capacity or take on an activity not experienced in. It is evident from UKCC disciplinary hearings and anecdotal evidence that some nurses succumb. The nurses may genuinely believe they are competent to carry out the activities, but it might sometimes be due to pressure or being flattered at being asked. Many nurses do accept responsibility beyond their limits and at times do not appreciate that they will be held accountable. The buck stops with the nurse who accepts the responsibility and carries out the task; she has said I fully understand and know how to do this task.

If a nurse in primary care accepts the responsibility from a doctor to undertake screening activities for instance, without the required qualification, knowledge and experience, she is denying the general practitioner the right for his practice to meet the required standards. She is also failing in her duty of care and putting patients and clients at risk. As nurses understand and take on board the ramifications of clinical governance and the incumbent responsibility and accountability it espouses, they will no doubt embrace the implications of their practice for client outcomes and ultimately professional judgement. Newton (1999) explains how wound care can be improved through clinical governance. Clinical governance is intended to improve both clinical performance and professional practice by setting clear policies for clinical care and by monitoring compliance with these.

The Law

Of major importance to the nurse is case law. The law of tort is part of the old unwritten common law and has been interpreted and clarified over the years through the court system. It is therefore often seen to be 'judge made', as the findings of judges in the higher courts become binding on later similar cases (Padfield, 1983). Two torts – negligence and trespass – have a major influence on nurses behaviour. Modification of case law is dependent to some extent on the use of expert witnesses to inform the court of what is accepted professional practice in the particular circumstances of the case. This is one way in which judges can be informed of changes in practice so that law can be amended. Case law is also needed to interpret statute law. Statutes are usually drawn up to legislate over a broad range of circumstances and can never be worded in sufficient detail to answer every query that arises.

The law is slow to change in response to social developments. Bills are often pushed through parliament quickly when the government supports legislative change. Those changes/issues not promoted by government are reliant on a Member of Parliament putting forward a Private Members Bill.

Negligence

The tort of negligence has a major influence on nurses' practice. For negligence, there must be a duty of care, a failure in that duty and resultant harm (Padfield, 1983). A key issue is the definition of what standard of care the law requires. 'The medical standard of care is the standard of a reasonably skilled experienced doctor' (Bolam *v* Friern, HMC 1957), and this concept of reasonableness applies to any professional in any situation.

Harm can come from a number of nursing actions for example; a patient breaks a limb. Is there negligence or not? The answer has to relate back to the reasonableness of the standard of care at the time. If the patient were confused or disorientated, close observation and precautionary measures would be expected, but not if the patient had previously been alert and physically stable. This is where it is important for sufficiently detailed nursing records to demonstrate what care was given and its appropriateness. Any unusual circumstances must be recorded as these may have an effect on the standard of care that could be expected in the particular situation (UKCC, 1998). The nurse can also bring harm to the patient if they have not ensured that the patient is adequately informed about the progress of their disease or risks of certain treatments.

Patients are entitled to choice and decision making regarding their care. A problem may exist in recognizing one's own limitations. The inexperienced may not realise some of the potentially serious implications of performing certain functions inadequately. However, the law is clear on the responsibilities of those concerned. The Wilsher case (Wilsher *v* Essex, AHA 1986–88) highlighted the point that inexperience can never be an excuse. The duty of care required by law is that expected of the post not the post-holder (Tingle, 1989). It is, therefore, the responsibility of a nurse, if inexperienced in a particular type of care to check her competence carefully and if necessary ask for training. The nurse will need to consider if it is in the patient's interest to adapt her role in the way suggested, good standards of care may be jeopardised if additional resources are not made to support such activities. For instance, nurse led clinics and counselling services.

There is sometimes difficulty in ascertaining the boundaries of practice and where ultimate responsibility lies. Nurses may take on an increased/enhanced role because she is acting as an independent practitioner. However, the task undertaken may have been delegated as one previously undertaken by a medical practitioner. The GMC has offered doctors guidance on this. The (GMC) (1995) states that:

> ... You may delegate medical care to nurses and other health care staff who are not registered medical practitioners if you believe it is best for the patient. However, you must be sure that the person to whom you delegated is competent to undertake the procedure or therapy involved. When delegating care or treatment, you just always pass on enough information about the patient and the treatment needed. You will still be responsible for managing the patient's care.

Where tasks are delegated, then the doctor delegating the task should follow appropriate guidelines (General Medical Council, 1995 p. 9).

Nurse Prescribing

Following the Crown Report (Department of Health, 1999) nurses now have an opportunity to expand their role even further. In 1986, the Cumberlage report stated that community nurses should have prescribing rights. In 1992, legislation was introduced in the form of Medicinal Products (Prescription by Nurses) Act. There has been much debate and uncertainty of the outcome of nurse prescribing. The final Crown report recommended the following:

- the majority of patients continue to receive medicines on an individual patient specific basis;
- the current prescribing authority of doctors, dentists and certain nurses (in respect of a limited list of medicines) continues;
- new groups of professionals would be able to apply for authority to prescribe in specific clinical areas, where this would improve patient care and patient safety could be assured.

The report also recommends distinguishing between categories of pre-scribers:

(i)   Independent prescribers – are professionals who are responsible for the initial assessment of the patient and for devising the broad treat-ment plan, with the authority to prescribe the medicines required.

(ii) Dependent prescribers – professionals who are authorised to pre-scribe medicines for patients whose condition has been diagnosed or assessed by an independent prescriber, within an agreed assessment and treatment plan (Department of Health, 1999).

Where nurses act as prescribers they must ensure that they are acting within the powers given by statute. When the nurse is prescribing drugs, she will be judged by the standard of the experienced nurse undertaking such a role. If nurses are involved in prescribing drugs, they must check the dose given; negligent prescription of an overdose may lead to an action of negligence (Dwyer *v* Roderick 1983, 127SJ801), as may writing an illegible prescription (Prendagast *v* Sam and Dee, *The Times* (1989) and I. Med CR 36). Developments in nursing practice may result in the increased possibility of litigation.

Consent

Much of the legal framework of patients' interests can be encompassed by the tort of trespass to the person. For example, assault and battery (in their civil law meaning). A major legal defence against an action for trespass is consent and an important concept here is capacity (Young, 1994).

> The capacity to give legally effective consent depends on the capacity to understand and come to a decision on what is involved and the capacity to communicate that decision. (Skegg, 1984 p. 151)

Gaining consent is often seen as being the business of doctors rather than nurses. For a number of reasons this can be disputed especially with the progress of nursing activities encompassed within the Scope of Practice.

The significance of the nurse's responsibility in relation to patient's interests is underpinned by the first statement of the Code of Professional Conduct. 'Safeguard and promote the interests of individual patients and clients.' (UKCC, 1992). Even legally, the nurse has a role to play in consent. Particularly as previously stated, the nurse takes on experiences of their role and creates new nursing initiatives. Consent can be implied, oral or written. It is usually assumed that the patient gives consent to nursing care, either orally or through acceptance of care being given. Nurses do, however, generally believe that patients/clients do give consent. In both theory and practice, nurses discuss issues related to individualised care, but in fact, if nurses scrutinised their actions, they may find that patients do not always exercise choice or take active roles in deciding the care they would like to receive.

Nurses do need to acknowledge their legal responsibility regarding consent, particularly if, as previously stated they are involved in some way with advanced technical skills undertaken by doctors or if for instance they are instrumental in developing a nurse led initiative. The nurse not choosing to expand her role may be unlikely to become involved in an action for battery, it is clear that she could be negligent if harm resulted from the giving of wrong information. For example, a practice nurse not fully informing a mother of the advantages and disadvantages of immunization for her child and the child receiving damage from the drug administered.

This is even more crucial for the nurse practitioner who may action diagnostic skills and prescribe medication for a client and resultant damage ensues. The nurse does have some responsibilities:

1. To clarify information given by a doctor, the patient may, because of anxiety misinterpret or mishear what is actually said by a doctor.

2. Secondary information may help the patient come to a decision, for example the type of nursing care (Young, 1994).

3. The nurse may wish to give additional medical information, but she needs to be sure of the facts as the doctor is usually in control of the medical information given.

4. The nurse also has a responsibility as an advocate for the patient (UKCC, 1992). Helping the patient to formulate and then ask appropriate questions of the doctor. Having a nurse do this may give the patient confidence in doing this. The nurse may also be in a position to enlarge on what is being said. The consent form suggested by the NHS Executive states that the patient might ask for a relative, friend or a nurse to be present (NHS Executive, 1990).

It can be seen that at a legal level, there is a dilemma in the legal stance related to negligence and its relationship to battery. Negligence with its basis in the duty of care emphasizes the need to act in accordance with safeguarding the well-being of the individual. Balancing patient rights and duties is often difficult. A failure to act might be construed as negligence as might overriding patients wishes.

The argument that if professionals act in the best interests of the patients this will provide protection against legal actions is unlikely to be infallible and the nurse may in fact have little voice in some of the decisions on what is in the patient's best interest. There are other conflicts, at an employment level rocking the boat or whistle blowing prevents one from voicing an opinion when unemployment is high and jobs are valuable – with mortgages to pay and families to feed. Nurses have to balance their professional accountability, accountability to the employer, self and the public.

Protocols for Good Nursing Practice

Protocols have been established in Chapter 12 as an integral part of nurse led initiatives. They are used to assist diagnosis, to improve care, manage resources and for legal protection. Protocols can perform a useful function in achieving consensus and consistency in clinical practice between healthcare professionals for example the GP and the practice nurse who are working independently in the care of the same patient.

It is advantageous to the nurse to set out in writing a sequence of activities, particularly as work becomes more complex and specialized, or where role functions have changed. When using protocols it is advisable that:

- the purpose of the protocol is explicit
- it is founded on research based evidence
- it is used to assist health professionals deal with complex situations
- all those who are to use it should produce it, the content is agreed and the protocol should be reviewed at any time (Manian, 1997).

Record Keeping

Record keeping is a vital part of the nurse's professional role and there are government directives and professional standards that have to be met. These include:

- the Patients Charter (Department of Health, 1996)
- the UKCC Guidelines for Record Keeping (UKCC, 1998)
- Data Protection Act (1984)
- access to Patient Records (Anon, 1992).

All records are potential legal documents and (Young and Tingle, 1995 p. 179) define records as: 'Records are any permanent form of information recorded about a patient or client.' Records include computer held records, patient assessment and care plans, evaluators of care, observation charts e.g. wound assessments and forms or books recording incidents such as, lifting, accidents, violence and near misses.

As stated earlier, all records are potential legal documents and may be called for use in court actions. Adequate records are essential for both civil and criminal cases if a fair hearing is to take place. Inadequate records may lead to the patient being given the benefit of the doubt and an award of damages against the nurse or employing authority. All patients, their relatives, or members of the public, a nurse or anyone who feels they should complain, have a right to lodge complaints with the Community Health Council or the Health Service Commissioner. The Health Service Commissioner is required to produce reports to parliament or complaints received, and the examination of complaints relies heavily on records being made, for instance, issues of abuse or annoyed relatives, should be reported to a line manager and recorded in an incident book. You may also be concerned about a situation and may wish to make your own personal records in the event of a complaint being made. If you are concerned about making permanent records consult a union representative or senior colleagues who will advise you.

The Limitation Act 1980 requires that an action for personal injuries and death (medical negligence) must be brought within three years of the date of the cause of action or when any damage became apparent to the sufferer. The exception to this is a child who has suffered personal injury where there is no time barrier until she reaches the age of 21 years.

The Access to Health Records Act 1990 allows a patient to request to see his/her notes. Permission can only be withheld if the doctor considers that to do so would be harmful to the patient's physical or mental health. Similar rights exist under the Data Protection Act 1984 for information held on computer.

Nurses in all settings need to review their record keeping. However, in areas such as GP practices all those involved in record keeping need to develop an audit tool to ensure accurate and legal documentation.

Product Endorsement

It is recognized that in today's climate nurses may be asked to endorse pharmaceutical products. In addition, the nurse may be expected to work collaboratively with other healthcare practitioners in the endorsement. Before endorsing products, the nurse has to consider several issues:

- responsibility to the client
- responsibility to the profession

- responsibility to the employer
- responsibility to the public at large (society)
- responsibility to researchers and scientists
- responsibility to self.

There are several major issues related to product endorsement. Accountability, consent, advocacy, the legal stance, particularly duty of care and prevention of corruption.

The Code of Conduct is clear on the nurse's responsibilities:

> As a registered nurse … you must 'ensure that your registration status is not used in the promotion of commercial products or services, declare any financial or other interests in relevant organisations providing such goods or services and ensure that your professional judgement is not influenced by any commercial considerations. (UKCC, 1992)

The nurse needs to remember that at no time should the patient's freedom of choice or the nurse's professional judgement be compromised.

The terms of any sponsorship contract, which are within the statutory powers of the Health Authority, must be arrived at by tender or negotiation. Once met such contracts are subject to ordinary law of contract. Health Authorities need:

1. to take precautions to ascertain the standing of the sponsor
2. be aware of the Prevention of Corruption Act 1889–1916
3. be aware of Rule 16 UKCC Code of Professional Conduct
4. be aware of the sections on Advertising and Sponsorship in UKCC Guidelines for Professional Practice (UKCC 1996) para. 70–8.

Companies sometimes offer funding for some posts, projects or services, some of which have a commercial interest in matters associated with health care. Sponsorship arrangements that affect the professional judgement of registered practitioners should be brought to the attention of those who provide healthcare 'services'. The nurse is reminded of three major issues: consent; advocacy; and accountability.

Advocacy

Ethical issues for consideration for the nurse are among the following:

- product endorsement may impinge on the professional judgement of a nurse

- product endorsement may impinge unfavourably on the choice of goods for patients
- sponsorship/endorsement of a product may inhibit research and development of new/other products
- the nurse may become compromized
- a monopoly position in the market place may arise, reducing choice and possible higher costs.

The nurse, therefore, has many responsibilities. To always work in the best interests of the client. She should have a sound knowledge of the product and of others, and inform the client of *all* the options.

The nurse should refuse to endorse a product if it may not be to benefit the client. The nurse should also be aware of her contract of employment and not undertake to endorse a product outside of the employers contract. Many drug companies offer inducements for support of their products. Therefore, the nurse needs to be aware that she would be in breach of the Code of Conduct if she received goods or money in exchange for endorsement of a product.

Conclusion

This chapter has highlighted some particular professional issues related to primary care nursing. It is evident that nurses need to be vigilant in recognizing their accountability, especially as roles change through development and innovation guided by the Scope of Practice. Nurses working alone or in collaboration with other health workers need to heed their ethico-legal responsibilities as they move into nurse prescribing, endorsing medical products and working independently as practitioners in nurse led clinics.

The rapidly expanding scope of the practice nurse role has allowed opportunity for the development of many exciting nurse-led initiatives over recent years The primary care nurse needs to remain aware of the potential pitfalls as highlighted in this chapter. However, the judicious use of protocols, being familiar with the many and varied documents designed to protect nurses along with adequate training should endeavour to promote safe practice and a professional service to clients. In particular, due to the increased autonomy found in chronic disease management, nurses need to pay attention to each aspect of professional accountability – accountability to oneself, the public and one's employer – in order to find a balance between the demands of an increased scope of practice and being safe in that practice.

Appendix

Further Resources

A comprehensive site for all UK government publications can be found at
http://www.open.gov.uk/
Health pages in particular can be found at
http://www.open.gov.uk/index/thealth.htm

Asthma

National Asthma Campaign
   Providence House, Providence Place, London N1 ONT
   Tel: 0171 226 2260
NAC Asthma Helpline: 03450 10203 and 08457 10203
British Lung Foundation
   78 Hatton Garden, London, EC1N 8JR
   Tel: 0171 831 5831
   www.asthma.org.uk/page1.html

Training Courses

National Asthma and Respiratory Training Centre
   The Athenaeum, 10 Church Street, Warwick, CV34 4AB
   Tel: 01926 493313
   www.nartc.org.uk
The Asthma Management Centre
   232 Tower Street, Brunswick Business Park, Liverpool, L3 4BJ
   Tel: 0151 707 1141.

Diabetes

Diabetes UK (formerly British Diabetic Association)
   10 Queen Ann Street, London, W1M 0BD
   Tel: 0171 323 1531; 0800 60 70 60
   www.diabetes.org.uk/diabuk/frame/diabuk
Diabetes UK Life Assurance Quoteline: 0161 829 5600
Diabetes UK Travel Quoteline: 0171 512 0890
Diabetes Insight *http://www.diabetic.org.uk/*

Training Courses

The Diabetes Training Centre
  4 Station Road, Esholt, Shipley, West Yorkshire, BD17 7QR
  Tel: 01943 877388
ENB 928 Courses in Diabetes available through local Nurse Training Centres:
  The Manchester Diabetes Centre
  130 Hathersage Road, Manchester, MB 0HZ
  Tel: 0161 276700
Hypertension/CHD:
British Heart Foundation *www.bhf.org.uk*
Coronary Prevention Group *www.healthpro.org.uk*
Information on protocols and research:
British Hypertension Society *http://www.hyp.ac.uk/bhs/*

Training Courses

The British Hypertension Society Information Service Tel: 0181 725 3412 (advises on local courses on hypertension and CHD risk factors)
Making it Happen: British Heart Foundation: Heart Save Project Tel: 0186 522 6975 (a course based on evidence and designed to promote good practice)
Coronary Heart Disease Prevention in Primary Care
  The Diabetes Training Centre, 4 Station Road, Esholt. Shipley, West Yorkshire, BD17 7QR
  Tel: 01943 877388.

Epilepsy

British Epilepsy Association
  Anstey House, 40 Hanover Square, Leeds, LS3 1BE
  Tel: 0113 243 9393
  Freephone Helpline: 0800 30 90 30
BEA Website *www.epilepsy.org.uk*

Further Reading

Chadwick, D. (1997) *The encyclopaedia of epilepsy* Maghull, and Merseyside: Roby Education Ltd.
Taylor, M. (1996) *Managing epilepsy in primary care*. Blackwell Science, Oxford
Sander, J. W. and Y. M. Hart (1997) *Epilepsy: Questions and answers*. Merit Publishing International, Basingstoke.

Training Courses

Professional Diploma in Epilepsy Care
  Jane Buckingham/Professor C. G. Beddow, Faculty of Health and
  Environment, Leeds Metropolitan University, LS1 3HE
ENB N45 Epilepsy Care
  British Epilepsy Association
  Anstey House, 40 Hanover Square,
  Leeds, LS3 1BE
National Society of Epilepsy
  Chesham Lane, Chalfont St Peter, Gerrards Cross, Bucks, SL9 0RJ.

Others

DVLA (Driver and Vehicle Licensing Agency)
  Drivers Medical Unit, Longview Road, Morriston, Swansea, SA99 ITU
Emergency Identification System
  MedicAlert, 12 Bridge Wharf, 156 Caledonian Road, London, N1 9UU
  Tel: 0171 833 3034

Royal National Institute for the Blind
  224 Great Portland Street, London, W1N 6AA
  Tel: 0171 388 1266

Smoking Cessation
  Quit, Victory House, 170 Tottenham Court Road, London, W1P OHA
  Tel: 0171 388 5775
  Quitline Free 24 hour helpline for patients: 0800 00 22 00.

Bibliography

Agertoft, L. and S. Pederson (1994) 'Effects of long-term treatment with an inhaled corticosteroid on growth and pulmonary function in asthmatic children'. *Respiratory Medicine.* 88: 373–8.

Agrawal, B., A. Berger, K. Wolf and F.C. Luft (1996) 'Microalbuminuria screening by reagent strip predicts cardiovascular risk in hypertension'. *Journal of Hypertension.* 14(2): 223–8.

Aizawa, H., T. Iwanaga, H. Inoue, S. Takata and K. Matsumoto (2000) Once daily theophylline reduces serumeosinophil cationic protein and eosinophil levels in induced sputum of asthmatics. *International Archives of Allergy and Immunology.* February 121(2): 123.

Alberti, K.G. (1999) 'A desktop guide to Type 2 diabetes mellitus. European Diabetes Policy Group'. *Exp Clin Endocrinol Diabetes.* 107(7): 390–420.

Alberti, K.G. and P.Z. Zimmer (1998) 'Definition, diagnosis and classification of diabetes mellitus and its complications. Part 1: diagnosis and classification of diabetes mellitus. Provisional report of the World Health Organisation consultation'. *Diabetic Medicine.* 15: 539–53.

Alderman, M.H. (1994) 'Non-pharmacological treatment of hypertension'. *Lancet.* 344: 307–11.

Altura, B.M. and B.T. Altura (1995) 'Magnesium in cardiovascular biology'. *Scientific American Science and Medicine.* 2(3): 28–37.

Amiel, S.A. (1993) 'Hypoglycaemia in diabetes mellitus'. *Medicine International.* 21(7): 279–81.

Anon (1992) 'Access to Patient Records'. *Nursing Standard.* 22 July 6: 32.

Anon (1995) 'Prescription cost deters drug uptake'. *Nursing Times.* 91(26): 8.

Anon (1996) 'Adult blood pressure screening'. *Nurse Practitioner: American Journal of Primary Health Care.* 21(2): 112–16.

Appleton, M. and L. Jerreat (1995) 'Hypoglycaemia'. *Nursing Standard.* October 25–31, 10(5): 36–40.

Asch, S.E. (1956) 'Studies of independence and conformity: A minority of one against a unanimous majority'. *Psychological Monographs.* 70: 416.

Ausburn, L. (1981) 'Patient compliance with medication regimes'. In J.L. Sheppard (ed.) *Advances in Behavioural Medicine*: Vol. 1. Cumberland College, Sidney, Australia.

Barker, D.J.P., A.R. Bull, G. Osmond and S.J. Simmonds (1990) 'Fetal and placental size and risk of hypertension in adult life'. *British Medical Journal.* 301: 259–62.

Barnes, P.J. and S. Godfrey (1995) *Asthma.* Martin Dunitz Ltd, London.

Barnett, A. (1994) 'A significant risk'. *Nursing Times.* 90(2): 60–4.

Barry, P.W. and C. O'Callaghan (1996) 'Inhalational drug delivery from seven different spacers'. *Thorax.* 51: 835–40.

Barry, P.W., C. Robertson and C. O'Callaghan (1993) 'Optimum use of a spacer device'. *Archives of Diseases in Childhood.* 69: 693–4.

Beasley, R., W.R. Roche, J.A. Roberts and S.T. Holgate (1989) 'Cellular Events in the Bronchi in mild asthma and after Bronchial Provocation'. *American Review of Respiratory Disease* 139: 806–17.

Beauchamp, T.L. and J.F. Childress (1989) *Principles of Biomedical Ethics.* 3rd edn Oxford University Press, Oxford.

Beevers, D.G. and G.A. MacGregor (1988) *Hypertension in Practice.* Dunitz: London.

Beevers, D.G. and G.A. MacGregor (1995) *Hypertension in Practice.* 2nd edn Martin Dunitz, London.

Benner, P. (1984) *From Novice to Expert – Excellence and Power in Clinical Nursing Practice*, Addison Wesley Publishing Co., Menlo Park, California.

Bennet, N.E. (1994) 'Hypertension in the elderly'. *Lancet.* 34(820): 447–9.

Benzeval, M., K. Judge and M. Whitehead (eds) (1995) *Tackling Inequalities in Health: An agenda for Action.* Kings Fund, London.

Bingley, P.J. and E.A.M. Gale (1993) 'Aetiology and pathology of diabetes'. *Medicine International.* 21(7): 239–41.

Bion, W.R. (1961) *Experiences in Groups and Other Papers,* Tavistock Publications, London.

Bishop, A.H. and J.R. Scudder Jr. (1990) *The practical, moral and personal sense of nursing: a phenomenological philosophy of practice.* University of New York Press, Albany, New York State.

Boulton, A.J.M. (1993) 'The diabetic foot'. *Medicine International.* 21(7): 271–4.

Bousquet, J., P. Chanez and J.Y. Lacoste (1990) 'Eosonophilic inflammation in asthma'. *New England Journal of Medicine.* 323: 1033–9.

Bousquet, J. and F.B. Miches (1992) 'International Consensus Report on diagnosis and Management of Asthma'. *Allergy.* April, 47(2 part 2): 129–32.

Bowling, A. (1992) *Measuring Health: A Review of Quality of Life Measurements Scales.* Open University Press, Buckingham.

Boyce, N. (1998) 'Healing hearts'. *New Scientist.* November 21, 160(2161): 21.

Brazier, M. (1987) *Medicine, Patients and the Law.* Penguin, Harmondsworth.

Briggs, A. (1972) *Report on the Committee of Nursing,* Cmnd 5115, HMSO, London.

British Hypertension Society (1999) http://www.hyp.ac.uk/bhs/riskpv.htm accessed in August 2000.

British Thoracic Association (1992) 'Death from asthma in two regions of England'. *British Medical Journal.* 285: 1251–5.

Brooking, J. (1991) 'Doctors and Nurses: a personal view'. *Nursing Standard.* 11 December 6(12): 24–8.

Brown, A.M. (1998) 'Diabetes mellitus (1) The disease'. *The Pharmaceutical Journal.* 260: 704–6.

Brown, A.M. (1998a) 'Diabetes mellitus (2) Management of insulin-dependent diabetes mellitus'. *The Pharmaceutical Journal.* 260: 753–6.

Brown, A.M. (1998b) 'Diabetes mellitus (3) Management of non-insulin-dependent diabetes mellitus'. *The Pharmaceutical Journal.* 260: 905–8.

Brown, A.M. (1998c) 'Diabetes mellitus (4) Complications of diabetes: prevention and management'. *The Pharmaceutical Journal.* 261: 31–3.

Brown, F. (1996) 'Improving compliance with asthma therapy'. *Community Nurse.* 1(12): 30–1.

Brown, F. (1997) 'Patient empowerment through education'. *Professional Nurse Study Supplement.* 13(3): S4–S6.

Brown, S., T. Betts, D. Chadwick, B. Hall, S. Shorvon and S. Wallace (1993) 'An epilepsy needs document'. *Seizure:* 2(2) July: 91–103.

BTS (1997) 'The British Guidelines on Asthma Management. The 1995 Review and Position Statement'. *Throax.* Supplement: S1–2.

Buck, D., A. Jacoby, G.A. Baker, S. Graham-Jones and D.W. Chadwick (1996) 'Patients' experiences of and satisfaction with care for their epilepsy'. *Epilepsia.* 37(9) September: 841–9.

Burnard, P. (1995) *Learning Human Skills, An Experiential and Reflective Guide for Nurses.* Butterworth-Heinneman, Oxford.

Burr, M.L. (1995) 'Pollution: does it cause asthma?'. *Archives of Diseases in Childhood.* 72: 377–87.

Bury, T. and J. Mead (1998) *Evidence based healthcare. A practical guide for therapists.* Butterworth-Heinemann, Oxford.

Cameron, K. and F. Gregor (1987) 'Chronic illness and compliance'. *Journal of Advanced Nursing.* 12(6): 671–6.

Campbell, D.A., P.M. Yellowlees, G. McLennan and J.R. Coates (1995) 'Psychiatric and Medical Features of new fatal asthma'. *Thorax.* 50: 204–59.

Campbell, N., J. Thain, H. Deans, L. Ritchie, M. Rawles and J. Squair (1998) 'Secondary prevention clinics for coronary heart disease: randomised'. *British Medical Journal.* 9 May, 316(7142): 1434–7.

Cantrill, J. (1997) 'Tablets for diabetes – a quick reference guide'. *Diabetic Nursing.* 25.

Carroll, R. (1994) 'Kidney damage in diabetes'. *Nursing.* 5(6): 17–19.

Carvalho, J.J.M., R.G. Baruzzi, P.F. Howard, N. Poulter, M.P. Alpers, L.J. Franco, L.F. Marcopito, V.J. Spooner, A.R. Dyer, P. Elliott, P. Stamler and R.l. Stamler (1989) Blood pressure in four remote populations in the Intersalt Study. *Hypertension.* 14: 238–46.

Chang, A.B., P.D. Phelan, J.B. Carlin, S.M. Sawyer and C.F. Robertson (1998) 'A randomised, placebo controlled trial of inhaled salbutamol and beclomethasone for recurrent cough'. *Archives of Disease in Childhood.* 79: 6–11.

Chaplin, J., R.Y. Lasso, S. Shorvon and M. Floyd (1992) 'National general practice study of epilepsy: the social and psychological effects of a recent diagnosis of epilepsy'. *British Medical Journal*. May 6839(304): 1416–18.

Chappell, B. (1992) 'Epilepsy: patient views on their condition and treatment'. *Seizure*. 1 June (2) 103–109.

Charles, H. (1996) 'Developing a leg ulcer management programme'. *Professional Nurse*. 11(7): 475–7.

Charlton, I.,G. Charlton, J. Broomfield and M.A. Mullee (1990) 'Evaluation of peak flow and symptoms only self management plans for control of asthma in general practice'. *British Medical Journal*. 301: 1355–9.

Chatellier, G. and J. Menard (1997) 'The absolute risk as a guide to influence the treatment decision-making process in mild hypertension'. *Journal of Hypertension*. 15(3): 217–19.

Cochrane, A.L. and W.W. Holland (1971) 'Validation of screening procedures'. *British Medical Bulletin*. 27: 3–8.

Cochrane, G.M.W. Jackson and P.J. Rees (1996) *Asthma: Current Perspectives*. Mosby-Wolfe, London.

Cockerell, O.C., A.L. Johnson, J.W.A.S. Sander, Y.M. Hart, D.M.G. Goodridge and S. Shorvon (1994) 'Mortality from epilepsy: results from a prospective population based study'. *Lancet*. 2 October (344) 918–21.

Collins, R., R. Peto, J. Godwin and S. MacMahon (1990) 'Blood pressure and coronary heart disease'. *Lancet*. 336: 370–1.

Conceicao, S., M.K. Ward and D.N.S. Kerr (1976) 'Defects in sphygmomanometers: an important source of error in blood pressure recording'. *British Medical Journal*. 1: 886–8.

Cook, P.J., P. Davies, D.G. Beeves, R. Wise and D. Honeybourne (1998) '*Chlamydia pneumoniae* antibodies in severe essential hypertension'. *Hypertension*. 31(2): 589–94.

Coon, D. (1983) *Introduction to Psychology. Exploration and Application*. 3rd edn. West Publishing Company, New York.

Cooper, R.S., C.N. Rotimi and R. Ward (1999) 'The puzzle of hypertension in African-Americans'. *Scientific American*. 280(2): 36–43.

Crompton, G.K. (1988) 'Problems patients have using pressurised aerosol inhalers'. *European Journal of Respiratory Diseases*. 63 (Suppl 119): 101–4.

Crompton, G. (1998) *Respiratory Disase: Simplifying the approach*. A report from a Peer Review Panel, Medeva Pharma Ltd, Oxford.

Cross, S., S. Buck and J. Hubbard (1998) 'ABC of allergies: Allergy in general practice'. *British Medical Journal*. 316: 1584–7.

Cutler, J.A., D. Follmann P. Elliott and Suh II (1991) 'An overview of randomized trials of sodium reduction and blood pressure'. *Hypertension*. 17(Supplement I): I27–33.

Dahlof, B., L.H. Lindholm, L. Hansson, B. Schersten, T. Ekbom and P.-O. Wester (1991) 'Morbidity and mortality in the Swedish trial in old patients with hypertension (Stop-Hypertension)'. *Lancet*. 338(8778): 1281–4.

Davies, C. (1996) 'Cloaked in a tattered illusion … professionalism'. *Nursing Times*, 92(45): 44–6.

Dawkins, J.L., P.M. Crawford and T.G. Stammers (1993) 'Epilepsy: a general practice study of knowledge and attitudes among sufferers and non-sufferers'. *British Journal of General Practice*. 43(376): 1028–30.

Department of Health (1984) *Data Protection Act*. Department of Health, HMSO.

Department of Health (1988) *Promoting Better Health*. HMSO: London.

Department of Health (1989a) *A Strategy for nursing: A Report of the Steering Committee*. HMSO: London.

Department of Health (1989b) *Working for patients*. White Paper CM 555. HMSO: London.

Department of Health (1990) *The New GP Contract*. HMSO: London.

Department of Health (1991) *The Patients Charter*. HMSO: London.

Department of Health (1992) PL/CNO (92) 4. *The Extended Role of the Nurse. Scope of Professional Practice*. 19 June. Department of Health: London.

Department of Health (1992) *The Health of the Nation: A strategy for Health in* England. Cm1986 London: HMSO.

Department of Health (1993) *Report of the taskforce on the Strategy for Research in Nursing, Midwifery and Health Visiting*. HMSO: London.

Department of Health (1994) *Nutritional aspects of cardiovascular disease: A report of the Committee on Medical Aspects of Food Policy.* HMSO: London.

Department of Health (1996) *Choice and Opportunity: Primary Care – the future.* The Stationery Office: London.

Department of Health (1996) *Primary care: Delivering the Future.* The Stationery Office: London.

Department of Health (1996) *The National Health Service: A Service with Ambitions.* The Stationery Office: London.

Department of Health (1997) *Practice Nursing – a changing role to meet changing needs.* HMSO: London.

Department of Health (1997) *The New NHS, Modern, Dependable.* The Stationery Office: London.

Department of Health (1998) *A first class service, quality in the NHS.* The Stationery Office: London.

Department of Health (1998b) *Our Healthier Nation.* The Stationery office: London.

Department of Health (1999) *Health Act,* The Stationery Office: London.

Department of Health (1999) *Review of prescribing, supply, and administration of medicines. Final report* (Crown Report) March. http://www.doh.gov.uk/prescrib.htm

Derkx, F.H.M. and M.A.D.H. Schalekamp (1994) 'Renal artery stenosis and hypertension'. *Lancet.* 344: 237–9.

DHSS (1980) *Inequalities in Health: Report of a research working group* chaired by Sir Dougles Black. HMSO: London.

DHSS (1987) *Promoting Better Health.* HMSO: London.

Diabetes Control and Complications Research Group (1993) 'The effect of intensive treatment of diabetes on the development and progression of long-term complications in insulin-dependent diabetes mellitus'. *New England Journal of Medicine.* 329: 977–86.

Dickerson, J.E.C. and M.J. Brown (1995) 'Influence of age on general practitioners' definition and treatment of hypertension'. *British Medical Journal.* 310: 574.

Dickinson, J., S. Hutton, A. Artkin and K. Jones (1997) 'Reducing asthma morbidity in the community: the effect of a targeted nurse-run clinic in an English general practice'. *Respiratory Medicine.* 91: 634–40.

Douglas, E., M. Bennie, J. McAnaw and S. Hudson (1998) 'Pharmaceutical care. (4) Diabetes mellitus'. *The Pharmaceutical Journal.* 261: 810–18.

Draper, P. (1987) 'Not a job for juniors'. *Nursing Times.* 11 March, 83: 58–62.

Draper, P. (ed.) (1991) *Health through Public Policy: The greening of Public health.* Green Print: London.

Duff, L., A. Kitson, K. Seers and D. Humphris (1996) 'Clinical guidelines: an introduction to their development and implementation'. *Journal of Advanced Nursing.* 23(5): 887–95.

Dukes, J. and R. Stewart (1993) 'Be prepared'. *Health Service Journal.* 28 January 103: 24–5.

Duncan, C. (ed.) (2000) *MIMS,* Haymarket Press, London.

Duncan, J.S. and Y.M. Hart (1993) 'Medical Services'. In J. Laidlaw, A. Richens and D. Chadwick (eds). *A textbook of epilepsy.* Churchill Livingstone: Edinburgh.

Eddins, B. (1985) 'Chronic self-destructiveness as manifested by non-compliance behaviour in the hemodialysis patient'. *Journal of Nephrology Nursing.* July/August: 194–9.

Edwards, S. (1997) 'Recording blood pressure'. *Professional Nurse Study Supplement.* 13(2): S8–S11.

Effective Health Care (1998) 'Cholesterol and Coronary Heart disease: screening and treatment.' *NHS Centre of Reviews and Dissemination.* 4(1): 1–15.

Elwes, R.D., J. Marshall, A. Beattle and P.K. Newman (1991) 'Epilepsy and employment. A community based survey in an area of high unemployment'. *Journal of Neurology, Neurosurgery and Psychiatry.* 54(3): 200–3.

Elwood, J.M. (1990) 'Screening programmes in disease control'. In J.J. McNeil, R.W.F. King, G.L. Jennings and J.W. Powles (eds) *A Textbook of Preventive Medicine.* Edward Arnold: London.

Eriksen, J.E. and E.M. Kohner (1993) 'Diabetic retinopathy'. *Medicine International.* 21(7): 266–71.

Ertl, P. (1992) 'How do you make your treatment decision?'. *Professional Nurse.* 7(8): 543–52.

Everard, M.L., S.R. Clark and A.D. Milner (1992) 'Drug delivery from holding chambers with attached facemask'. *Archives of Diseases in Childhood.* 67: 580–5.

Expert Committee on the Diagnosis and Classification of Diabetes Mellitus (1997) 'Report of the Expert Committee on the Diagnosis and Classification of Diabetes Mellitus'. *Diabetes Care.* 20: 1183–97.

Fletcher, R.H., S.W. Fletcher and E.H. Wagner (1998) *Clinical Epidemiology: the Essentials.* Williams & Wilkins: New York.

Forrest, P. (1986) *Breast Cancer Screening: Report to the Health Ministers of England, Wales, Scotland and Northern Ireland.* HMSO: London.

Foster, P. (1995) *Women and the Health Care Industry: An Unhealthy Relationship?* Open University Press, Buckingham.

Fry, T. (1998) 'Growth and asthma: regular height assessment is an essential part of managing childhood asthma'. *Asthma Journal.* 3(2): 74–6.

Fullard, E., G. Fowler and M. Gray (1987) 'Promoting prevention in primary care: controlled trial of low technology, low cost approach'. *British Medical Journal.* 25 April, 294: 1080–2.

Funnell, M.M. and P. McNitt (1988) 'Autonomic neuropathy. Diabetics' hidden foe'. *American Journal of Nursing.* 86(3): 266–70.

Funnell, M. M., R.M. Anderson and M.S. Arnold (1991) 'Empowerment: an idea whose time has come in diabetes education'. *Diabetes Educator.* 17: 37–41.

Garmondsway, G.N. (1969) *The Penguin English Dictionary.* 2nd edn Penguin: Harmondsworth.

Garrett, J., S. Williams, C. Wong and D. Holdaway (1998) 'Treatment of acute asthmatic exacerbations with an increased dose of inhaled steroid'. *Arch Dis Child.* 79: 12–17.

General Medical Council (1995) *Duties of a Doctor: Guidance from the General Medical council. Good Medical Practice.* GMC: London.

Gerard, M.J. and M. Frank-Stromburg (1998) 'Screening for prostatic cancer in asymptomatic men: Clinical, ethical and legal implications'. *Oncology Nurse Forum.* 25 October (9): 1561–9.

Gibbs, C.J. (1993) 'Hyperlipidaemia in diabetes mellitus'. *Practical Diabetes.* 10(6): 214–16.

Gielen, M.H., S.C. Van der Zee, J.H. Van Wijnnnnen, C.J. Van Steen and B. Brunekreef (1997) 'Acute effects of summer pollution on respiratory health of asthmatic children'. *American Journal of Respiratory and Critical Care Medicine.* 155(6): 2105–8.

Gilbert, N. (1997) 'Lifestyle Management: Diet'. In G.M. Lindsay and A. Gaw (eds) *Coronary Heart Disease Prevention.* Churchill Livingstone: Edinburgh.

Goguen, J.M. and R.G. Josse (1993) 'Management of diabetic ketoacidosis'. *Medicine International.* 21(7): 275–8.

Gordis, L. (1979) 'Conceptual and methodological problems in measuring patient compliance'. In R.B. Haynes, D.W. Taylor and D.J. Sackett (eds) *Compliance in Health Care.* John Hopkins University Press: Baltimore.

Gordon, R.D. (1994) 'Mineralcorticoid hypertension'. *Lancet.* 344: 240–3.

Greening, A.P., P. Wind, M. Northfield and G. Shaw (1994) 'Added salmeterol versus higher dose corticosteroid in asthma patients with symptoms on existing inhaled corticosteroid'. *Lancet.* 344: 219–24.

Grimley Evans, J. and G. Rose (1971) 'Hypertension'. *British Medical Bulletin.* 27: 37–42.

Gross, R. (1996) *Psychology: The Science of Mind and Behaviour.* Hodder and Stoughton: London.

Hates, C.N. (1994) 'The Pathogenesis of NIDDM'. *Dibetologia.* September 37, Supplement 2: 5162–8.

Hamel, L. and K. Oberle (1996) 'Cardiovascular risk screening for women'. *Clinical Nurse Specialist.* 10(6): 275–9.

Hamet, P. (1996) 'Cancer and hypertension'. *Hypertension.* 28: 321–4.

Harrap, S.B. (1994) 'Hypertension: genes versus environment'. *Lancet.* 344: 169–71.

Hayden, M., C. Penna and N. Buchanan (1992) 'Epilepsy: patient perceptions of their condition'. *Seizure.* 1: 191–7.

Haynes, R.B. (1979) 'Introduction'. In R.B. Haynes, D.W. Taylor and D.L. Sackett (eds) *Compliance in Health Care.* John Hopkins University Press: Baltimore.

He, J., M.J. Klag, P.K. Whelton, J.-Y. Chen, J.-P. Mo, M.-C. Qian and G.-Q. Mo (1991) 'Migration, blood pressure pattern and hypertension: the Yi Migrant Study'. *American Journal of Epidemiology.* 134(10): 1085–101.

Health Education Authority (1994) *The Balance of Good Health.* HEA: London.

Heron, J. (1989) *Six Category Intervention Analysis,* 3rd edn Human Potential Research Group, University of Surrey: Guildford.

Higgins, C. (1994b) 'Laboratory backup'. *Nursing Times.* 90(32): 44–8.

Higgins, C. (1995) 'Pathology testing of blood glucose levels'. *Nursing Times.* 18(91): 42–4.

Higgins, C. (1994) 'Blood and urine tests for diagnosis and monitoring of diabetes'. *British Journal of Nursing.* 3(17): 886–91.

Hilgard, E.R., R.L. Atkinson and R. Atkinson (1979) *Introduction to Psychology.* 7th edn. Harcourt Brace Jovanovich: New York.

Hill, C. and J. Woodcock (1949) *The National Health Service.* Christopher Johnson: London.

Hilton, S. (1990) 'An audit of inhaler technique among asthma patients of 34 general practitioners'. *British Journal General Practice.* 40(341): 505–6.

Hirst, M., K. Atkin and N. Lunt (1995) 'Variations on practice nursing: implications for family health care services authorities'. *Health and Social Care in the Community.* 3: 83–97.

Hokanson Hawks, J. (1992) 'Empowerment in nursing education: concept analysis and application to philosophy, learning and instruction'. *Journal of Advanced Nursing.* 17: 609–18.

Holgate, S.T. (1996) 'The inflammatory basis of asthma and its implications for drug treatment'. *Clinical and Experimental Allergy.* June 26 (Supplement 4): 1–4.

Horne, R. (1997) 'Representations of medication and treatment advances in theory and mesurement'. In J.K. Petrie and J. Weinman (eds) *Perceptions of Health and Illness: Current Research and Applications.* Harwood Academic: London.

Hoskins, G. (1998) 'The effect of a trained asthma nurse on patient outcomes within a General Practice'. *Asthma in General Practice.* 6(1): 3.

House, N. (1996) 'Patient compliance with leg ulcer treatment'. *Professional Nurse.* 12(1): 33–6.

Houghton, M. and M. Whittow (1967) *Medical Nursing.* Balliere, Tindou & Cassell: London.

Iles, R., P. Lister, and A.T. Edmunds (1999) 'Crying significantly reduces the absorption of aerosolised drug in infants'. *Archives of Diseases in Childhood.* August 81(2): 163–5.

Institute of Medicine (1992) *Guidelines for clinical practice: from development to use.* National Academy Press: Washington DC.

Intersalt Cooperative Research Group (1988) 'Intersalt: an international study of electrolyte excretion and blood pressure. Results of 24 hour urinary sodium and potassium excretion'. *British Medical Journal.* 297(6644): 319–28.

Jacob, F. (1994) 'Ethics in health promotion: Freedom or determinism?' *British Journal of Nursing.* 3(6): 299–302.

Jacoby, A. (1993) 'Quality of life and care in epilepsy'. *Royal Society of Medicine Round Table series* 31. Oxford: Royal Society of Medicine, 66–73.

Jacques, A. (1993) 'The use of insulin in diabetes mellitus'. *Professional Nurse.* 9(3): 190–2.

Janis, I.L. and Mann, L. (1965). 'Effectiveness of emotional role-playing in modifying smoking habits and attitudes'. *Journal of Experimental Research in Personality.* 1: 84–90.

Jenkins, D. (1991) 'Investigations: how to get from guidelines to protocols'. *British Medical Journal* 303(6798): 323–33.

Johns, C. and D. Freshwater (1998) *Transforming Nursing Through Reflective Practice.* Blackwell Science: Oxford.

Joint National Committee on Prevention, Detection, Evaluation, and Treatment of High Blood Pressure (1997) *The sixth report of the Joint National Committee on Detection, Evaluation, and Treatment of High Blood Pressure.* National Institute of Health: Bethesda, MD.

Jones, M. (1995) *Whose Prescription.* RCN: London.

Jones, E. (1993) *Family Systems Therapy.* Wiley: Chichester.

Kaplan, N.M. (1994) 'Ethnic aspects of hypertension'. *Lancet.* 344: 450–2.

Kelly, J.C (1994) *Drug Compliance in Renal Patients.* (Unpublished MSc thesis.) University of Hertfordshire: Hertford.

Kelnar, C. (1996) *Childhood Growth, Practice Handbook.* Medicom, London.

Kemp, F., C. Foster and S. McKinlay (1993) 'Blood pressure measurement technique of clinical staff'. *Journal of Human Hypertension.* 7: 95–102.

Kiernan, V. (1996) 'Misplaced fears put patients off their pills'. *New Scientist.* 149(2022): 10.

King, J. (1984a) 'Psychology in nursing: striking it right'. Part 1. *Nursing Times.* 80(42): 29–31.

King, J. (1984b) 'Psychology in nursing: the health belief model'. *Nursing Times.* 80(43): 53–5.

Kingsworth, D. and S. Wilkinson (1996) 'Patient compliance with medication regimen after discharge from palliative care'. *International Journal of Palliative Care Nursing.* 2(3): 144–8.

Klatsky, A.L. (1995) 'Cardiovascular effects of alcohol'. *Scientific American Science and Medicine*. 2(2): 28–37.

Klatsky, A.L., G.D. Friedman, M.S. Siegelaub, and M.J. Gerard (1977) 'Alcohol consumption and blood pressure. Kaiser-Permanente multiphasic health examination data'. *New England Journal of Medicine*. 296: 1194–200.

Kuitert, L. (1999) 'Leukotriene receptor antagonists in clinical practice: has this new class of drugs for the treatment of asthma fulfilled its early promise?'. *The Asthma Journal*. 4(4): 154–6.

Kurtz, T.W (1994) 'Genetic models of hypertension'. *Lancet*. 344: 167–8.

Kyngas, H. and J. Barlow (1995) 'Diabetes: an adolescent's perspective'. *Journal of Advanced Nursing*. 22(5): 941–7.

Laitinen, L.A., M. Heino, A. Laitinen, T. Kava and T. Haahtela (1985) 'Damage of the airway epithelium and bronchial reactivity in patients with asthma'. *American Review of Respiratory Disease*. 131: 599–606.

Laitinen, L.A., A. Laitinen and T. Haahtela (1993) 'Airway Mucosal Inflammation Even in Patients with Newly Diagnosed Asthma'. *American Review of Respiratory Disease*. 147: 697–704.

Lakhani, S.R., S.A. Dilly and C.F. Finlayson (1993) *Basic Pathology: an Introduction to the Mechanisms of Disease*. Edward Arnold: London.

Lakin, V., T. Gill and W. Jones (1996) 'Diet and Coronary Heart Disease'. *Cardiology Update*. October 314–29.

Last, J.M. (ed.) (1988) *A dictionary of Epidemiology*. 2nd edn Oxford University Press: Oxford.

Law, M., N. Wald and S. Thompson (1994) 'By how much and how quickly does reduction in serum cholesterol concentration lower risk of IHD'. *British Medical Journal*. 308: 367–73.

Lawrence, R.D. (1960) *The diabetic ABC*. British Medical Journal Publishing Group: London.

Lee Tai S., M. Gold and S. Iliffe (1997) 'Promoting healthy exercise among older people in general practice: issues in designing and evaluating therapeutic interventions'. *British Journal of General Practice*. 47: 119–122.

Leestma, J.E., T. Walczak, J.R. Hughes, B.K. Mitra and S.T. Shaku (1989) 'A prospective study on sudden unexpected death in epilepsy'. *Annals of Neurology*. August 29(2) 195–203.

Levy, M., J. Couriel, R. Clark, S. Holgate and A. Chauhan (1997) *Shared care for Asthma Medical Media*. ISIS: Oxford.

Ley, P. (1988) 'The problem of patients' non-compliance'. In P. Ley (ed.) *Communicating with Patients – Improving Communication Satisfaction and Compliance*. Chapman & Hall: London.

Ley, P. and M.S. Spelman (1967) *Communicating with the Patient*. Staples Press, London.

Lindop, G.B.N. (1992) 'Hypertension'. In J. McGee, P. Isaacson and N.A. Wright (eds) *Oxford Textbook of Pathology. Volume 2a Pathology Of Systems*. University Press Oxford: Oxford.

Linjer, E. and L. Hansson (1997) 'Underestimation of the true benefits of antihypertensive treatment: an assessment of some important sources of error'. *Journal of Hypertension*. 15: 221–5.

Lipworth, B.J. (1999) 'Modern drug treatment of chronic asthma'. *British Medical Journal*. 318: 380–4.

Lowry, M. (1998) 'Clinical supervision for the development of nursing practice'. *British Journal of Nursing*. 7(9): 553–8.

Lupton, D. (1995) *The Imperative of Health: Public Health and the Regulated Body*. Sage: London.

MacKinnon, M. (1998) *Providing Diabetes Care in General Practice: A Practical guide for the Primary Care Team*. 3rd edn Class Publishing: London.

Macleod, A.F. (1993) 'Diabetic neuropathy'. *Medicine International*. 21(7): 261–3.

MacMahon, B. and T.F. Pugh (1970) *Epidemiology: Principles and Methods*. Little Brown & Co.: Boston.

MacMahon, S., R. Peto, J. Cutler, R. Collins, P. Sorlie, J. Neaton, R. Abbott, J. Godwin, A. Dyer and J. Stamler (1990) 'Blood pressure, stroke, and coronary heart disease. Part 1, prolonged differences in blood pressure: prospective observational studies corrected for the regression dilution bias'. *Lancet*. 335: 765–74.

Manian, R. (1997) 'Protocols and legal status'. *Care of the Critically Ill*. March/April 13(2): 44.

Markham, A. and D. Faulds (1998) 'Theophylline. A review of its potential steroid sparing effect in asthma'. *Drugs*. December 56(6): 1081–91.

Marshall, P. (1990) 'The heart as a gland'. *Nursing Times*. 86(7): 42–3.

McCowan, C., R.G. Neville, G.E. Thomas, I.K. Crombie, R.A. Clark, I.W. Ricketts, A.Y. Cairns, F.C. Warner, S.A. Greene and E. White (1998) 'Effect Of asthma and its treatment on growth: four year follow up of cohort of children from general practices in Tayside, Scotland'. *British Medical Journal*. 316: 668–72.

McGee, J., P. Isaacson and N.A. Wright (eds) (1992) *Oxford Textbook of Pathology. Volume 2a Pathology Of Systems.* University Press Oxford: Oxford.

McInnes, G. (1997) 'Anti-hypertensive therapy'. in G.M. Lindsay and A. Gaw (eds) *Coronary Heart Disease Prevention.* Churchill Livingstone: Edinburgh.

McLellan, A.R. (1993) 'Insulins'. *Medicine International.* 21(7): 250–1.

McLellan, A.R. (1993a) 'Oral hypoglycaemic agents'. *Medicine International.* 21(7): 255–6.

Medicines Resource Centre (1993) 'The treatment of hypertension in the elderly'. *MeReC Bulletin.* 4(9): 33–4.

Meichenbaum, D. and D.C. Turk (1987) *Facilitating Treatment Adherence – A Practitioner's Guidebook.* Plenum Press: London.

Menzies-Lyth, I. (1988) *The functioning of social systems as a defence against anxiety, in Containing Anxiety in Institutions, Selected Essays,* (Vol. 1), Free Association Books: London.

Millar, B. (1999) 'Carry that Weight', *Health Service Journal.* 18 February.

Mohan, G., B.D.W. Harrison, R.M. Badminton, S. Mildenhall and N.J. Wareham (1996) 'A confidential enquiry into deaths caused by asthma in an English health region: implications for general practice'. *British Journal General Practice.* 46: 529–32.

Moore, K.N. (1995) 'Compliance or collaboration? The meaning for the patient'. *Nursing Ethics: An International Journal for Health Care Professionals.* 2(1): 71–7.

Morrell, J. and J. Lynas (1998) 'Advising patients about diet and heart disease'. *Clinical Pulse.* March 14: 83–4.

Muncey, T. (2000) 'The Good Nurse: Born or Made?'. Unpublished Ph.D. *thesis.* Cranfield University: Beds.

Naidoo, J. and J. Wills (1994) *Health Promotion Foundations for Practice.* Balliere & Tindall: London.

National Asthma and Respiratory Training Centre (1999) *Devices under Discussion.* Direct Publishing Solutions: Berkshire.

National Asthma Campaign (1996) *The Impact of Asthma Survey. The effect of Asthma on Quality of Life.* Allen & Hanburys: London.

National Asthma Campaign (1999) 'Asthma Audit'. *Asthma Journal.* 32, December.

National Heart, Lung and Blood Institute (1992) 'International consensus report on the diagnosis and management of asthma'. *Clinical Exp Allergy.* (Supplement 1) 22: 1–72.

Neal, M.J. (1997) *Medical Pharmacology at a Glance.* 3rd edn Blackwell Science: Oxford.

Newman, S.P., D. Pavia and S.W. Clarke (1981) 'Deposition of pressurised aerosols in the human respiratory tracts'. *Thorax.* 36: 52–5.

Newton, H. (1999) 'Improving wound care through clinical governance'. *Nursing Standard.* 7 April, 13(29): 51–6.

NHS (1997) Primary Care Act. The Stationery Office: London.

NHS Executive (1990) *A guide to Consent for Examination or Treatment.* Department of Health: London.

NHS Executive (1999) *Clinical Governance: Quality in the new NHS.* Department of Health: London.

NHSE (1996) *Clinical Guidelines; using Clinical Guidelines to Improve Patient Care within the NHS.* Department of Health: London.

Nicolai, T. (1999) Environmental air pollution and lung disease in children. *Monaldi Arch Chest Dis.* December 54(6): 475–8.

Nightingale, F. (1860) *Notes on Nursing: What it is and What it is not.* Harrison: London.

North of England Evidence Based Guidelines Development Project (1996) 'Summary version of evidence based guidelines for the primary management of asthma in adults'. *British Medical Journal.* 312: 762–6.

Norton, D., R. McLaren and A.N. Exton Smith (1962) *An investigation of Geriatric Nursing in Hospital.* Churchill Livingstone: Edinburgh.

O'Brien, D. and M. Davison (1994) 'Blood pressure measurement: rational and ritual actions'. *British Journal of Nursing.* 3(8): 393–6.

O'Callaghan, C., J. Lynch, M. Cant and C. Robertson (1993) 'Improvement in sodium cromoglycate delivery from a spacer device by using an antistatic lining, immediate inhalation, and avoiding multiple actuations of drug'. *Thorax.* 48: 6,603–6.

O'Connor, B. (1996) 'How to select the most appropriate device for the adult asthmatic (a personal view)'. *Medical Dialogue.* 456.

O'Hanrahan, M. and K. O'Malley (1981) 'Compliance with drug therapy'. *British Medical Journal.* 283: 298–300.

Obholzer, A. and V.Z. Roberts (eds) (1994) *The Unconscious at Work, Individual and Organisational Stress in the Human Services* Routledge: London.

OPCS (1991) *Standard Occupational Classification.* Volume 3. HMSO: London.

Orchard, T. (1998) 'Diabetes: a time for excitement – and concern'. *British Medical Journal.* 317: 691–2.

Orem, D. (1991) *Nursing: concepts of practice.* 4th edn Mosby Year Book: St Louis.

Padfield, C. (1983) *Law Made Simple.* (Revised by F.E. Smith 6th edn). Heinemann: London

Paley, G. (1995) 'A framework for clinical protocols'. *Nursing Standard.* 15 February 9(21): 33–5.

Parkin, T. (1997) 'Patient control in dietary management'. *Professional Nurse Study Supplement.* 13(3): S7–S10.

Partridge, M.R. (1998) 'Difficult choices at Step 3'. *Asthma Journal.* 3(2): 58–9.

Paterson, J.R., A.R. Pettigrew and M.H. Dominiczak (1991) 'Screening for hyperlipidaemia in diabetes mellitus. Relationship to glycaemic control'. *Annals of Clinical Biochemistry.* 28: 354–8.

Pauwels, R.A., C.G. Lofdahl and D.S. Postma (1997) 'Effect of inhaled formoterol and budesonide on exacerbations of asthma'. *New England Journal of Medicine.* 337: 405–11.

Pearce, L. (1998) 'A Guide to Asthma Inhalers'. *Nursing Times Know How.* 4 March.

Pederson, S. (1987) 'Inhaler use in children with asthma'. *Danish Medical Bulletin.* 3: 234–49.

Petrie, J., M. Small and J. Connell (1997) '"Glitazones" a prospect for non-insulin-dependent diabetes'. *Lancet.* 349: 70–1.

Petrie, J.C., E.T. O'Brien, W.A. Littler and M. De Swiet (1986) 'British Hypertension Society: Recommendations on blood pressure measurement'. *British Medical Journal.* 293: 611–15.

Pfister-Minogue, K. (1993) 'Enhancing patient compliance: a guide for nurses'. *Geriatric Nursing.* 14(3): 124–32.

Pheley, A.M., P. Terry, L. Pietz, J. Fowles, C.E. McCoy and H. Smith (1995) 'Evaluation of a nurse-based hypertension management program: screening, management, and outcomes'. *Journal of Cardiovascular Nursing.* 9(2): 54–61.

Pickering, T.G. (1994) 'Blood pressure measurement and detection of hypertension'. *Lancet.* 344: 31–4.

Pickin, C. and S. St Leger (1993) *Assessing health needs using the life cycle framework.* Open University Press: Buckingham.

Pool, J. (1995) Personal Correspondence. Unpublished Data.

Postma, D.S., E.R. Bleeker and P.J. Amelung (1995) 'Genetic susceptibility to asthma bronchial hyper responsiveness co-inherited with a major gene for atopy'. *New England Journal of Medicine.* 333: 894–90.

Poulton, B. (1991) 'Factors improving compliance'. *Nursing Standard.* 5, 29 May. Supplement 3–5.

Prahl, P. and T. Jensen (1987) 'Decreased adrenocorticol suppression utilising the nebuhaler for inhalation of steroid aerosols'. *Clinical Allergy.* 17: 393–8.

Prochaska, J. and C.C. Diclemente (1984) *The Transtheroetical Approach: Crossing Traditional Foundations of Change.* Dan Jones: Irwin Homewood.

Psaty, B.M., S.R. Heckbert, T.D. Koepsell, D.S. Siscovick, T.E. Raghunathan, N.S. Weiss, F.R. Rosendaal, R.N. Lemaitre, N.L. Smith, P.W. Wahl, E.H. Wagner and C.D. Furberg (1995) 'The risk of myocardial infarction associated with antihypertensive therapies'. *Journal of the American Medical Association.* 274: 620–5.

Puddey, I.B., L.J. Beilin and R. Vandongen (1987) 'Regular alcohol use raises blood pressure in treated hypertensive subjects'. *Lancet.* I(8534): 647–51.

Ramsay, L.E., B. Williams, G.D. Johnston, G.A. MacGregror, L. Poston, J.F. Potter, N.R. Poulter and G. Russell (1999) 'BHS Guidelines: Guidelines for Management of Hypertension and Report of the Third Working Party of the British Hypertension Society'. *Journal of Human Hypertension.* 13: 569–92.

Raynor, D.K. (1991) 'Patient information and its influence on medication compliance'. Unpublished Ph.D. thesis. University of Bradford: Bradford.

Raynor, D.K. (1992) 'Patient compliance: the pharmacist's role'. *The International Journal of Pharmacy Practice.* March 126–35.

RCN (1992) *Diabetes Clinical Guidelines for Practice Nurses.* RCN: London.

REACH Primary Care Group (1998) *Who Owns Hypertension?* Merk, Sharpe & Dohrie Ltd: Herts.

Redington, A.E. and P.H. Howarth (1997) 'Airway Remodelling in Asthma'. *Thorax.* 52: 310–12.

Rees, J. and J. Price (1995) *ABC of Asthma.* 3rd edn. London: BMJ Publishing Group.

Reisin, E., R. Abel, M. Modan, D.S. Silverberg, H.E. Eliahou and B. Modan (1978) 'Effect of weight loss without salt restriction on the reduction of blood pressure in overweight hypertensive patients'. *The New England Journal of Medicine*. 298(1): 1–5.

Ridsdale, L., D. Robins, A. Fitzgerald, S. Jeffrey and L. McGee (1996) 'Epilepsy in general practice: Patients psychological symptoms and their perception of stigma'. *British Journal of General Practice*. June 46: 365–6.

Ridsdale, L., D. Robins, C. Cryer and H. Williams (1997) 'Feasibility and effects of nurse run clinics for patients with epilepsy in general practice: randomised controlled trial'. *British Medical Journal*. January 314(7074): 120–2.

Roberson, M. (1992). 'The meaning of compliance: patient perspectives'. *Qualitative Health Research*. 2(1): 7–26.

Roper, N. (1976) 'A model for nursing and nursology'. *Journal of Advanced Nursing*. 1: 219–27.

Rosenau, P.M. (1992) *Post-modernism and the Social Sciences*. Princeton University Press: Princeton, NJ.

Ross, F.M., P.J. Bower and B.S. Sibbald (1994) 'Practice Nurses, Workload and training needs'. *British Journal of General Practitioner*. 44: 15–18.

Sackett, D.L. and R.B. Haynes (eds) (1976) *Compliance with Therapeutic Regimens*. John Hopkins Press: Baltimore.

Sackett, D.L., W.M.O. Rosenburg, J.A.M. Gray, R.B. Liaynes and W.S. Richardson (1996) 'Evidence based medicine: what it is and what it isn't'. *British Medical Journal*. 312(7023): 71–2.

Salter, H.H. (1860) *On Asthma: its Pathology and Treatment*. J. Churchill: London.

Sampson, A. and S. Holgate (1998) 'Leukotriene modifiers in the treatment of asthma'. *British Medical Journal*. 316: 1257–8.

Sampson, A.P. (1996) 'The leukotrienes: mediators of chronic inflammation in allergy'. *Clinical and Experimental Allergy*. September; 26(9): 95–1004.

Sander, J.W. (1993) 'Some aspects of prognosis in the epilepsies'. *Epilepsia*. 34: 1007–116.

Sander, J.W.A.S. and S. Shorvon (1987) 'Incidence and prevalence studies in epilepsy and their methodological problems: a review'. *Journal of Neurology Neurosurgery and Psychiatry*. July 50(7): 829–39.

Sander, J.W.A.S. and S.D. Shorvon (1996) 'Epidemiology of the epilepsies'. *Journal of Neurology Neurosurgery and Psychiatry*. November 61(5): 433–43.

Scammell, B. (1990) *Communication Skills*. Macmillan: Basingstoke.

Sears, M.R., M.D. Holdaway, E.M. Flannery, G.P. Herbison and P.A. Silva (1996) 'Parental and neonatal risk factors for atopy, airway hyper-responsiveness, and asthma'. *Arch Dis Child*. 75: 392–8.

Seaton, E.D., M.A. Pinkney, D.P.J. Turner and J. Coady (1992) 'Pressurised metered dose inhaler technique; how good are general practitioners'. *Thorax*. 47: 237.

Sever, P., G. Beevers and C. Bulpitt, C. (1993) 'Management guidelines in essential hypertension: Report of the second working party of the Bristol Hypertension Society'. *British Medical Journal*. 306: 983–7.

Silverman, M. (1997) 'Wheeze in the under-fives'. *Paediatrics Update*. April, 550–6.

Sinclair, A.J. (1993) 'Rational approaches to the treatment of patients with non-insulin-dependent diabetes mellitus (NIDDM)'. *Practical Diabetes*. Supplement 10(6): S15–S20.

Skegg, P.D.G. (1984) *Law, Ethics and Medicine*. Oxford University Press: Oxford.

Slama, G. (1993) 'Insulin dependent diabetes mellitus'. *Medicine International*. 21(7): 252–5.

Soothill, K., L. Mackay and C. Webb (1995) *Interprofessional Relations in Healthcare*. Edward Arnold: London.

Staessen, J.A., G. Byttebier, F. Buntinx, H. Celis, E.T. O'Brien and R. Fagard (1997) 'Antihypertensive treatment based on conventional or ambulatory blood pressure measurement'. *Journal of American Medical Association*. 278(13): 1065–72.

Stalhofen, W., J. Gebbert and J. Heyder (1980) 'Experimental determination of the regional deposition of aerosol particles in the human respiratory tract'. *American Independent Hygiene Association Journal*. 41: 385.

Stevens, A. and J. Lowe (1995) *Pathology*. Mosby: London.

Stillwell, B. and A. Bowling (eds) (1996) *The Nurse in Family Practice: Practice Nurses & Nurse Practitioners in Primary Health Care*. Balliere Tindall: London.

Strandgaard, S. and O.B. Paulson (1994) 'Cerebrovascular consequences of hypertension'. *Lancet*. 344: 519–21.

Taylor, R.H. (1993) 'Post-prandial hyperglycaemia and diabetic complications'. *Practical Diabetes. Supplement* 10(6): S11–S14.

Taylor, M. (1987) 'Epilepsy in a Doncaster Practice: audit and change over eight years'. *Journal of Royal College of General Practice*. 37: 396–400.

Tettersell, M.J. (1993) 'Asthma patients' knowledge in relation to compliance with drug therapy'. *Journal of Advanced Nursing*. 18(1): 103–13.

Thapar, A. K. (1996) 'Care of patients with epilepsy in the community: will new initiatives address old problems?' *British Journal of General Practice*. January 46: (1402) 37–42.

The British Guidelines on Asthma Management (1997) *Thorax*. 52 (Supplement 1): S1–21.

The British Lung Foundation Inhaled Corticosteroids in Asthma. The Facts

The treatment of mild hypertension research group (1991) 'The treatment of mild hypertension study: A randomised placebo-controlled trial of a nutritional hygienic regimen along with various drug monotherapies'. *Archives of Internal Medicine*. 151: 1413–23.

Tingle, J.H. (1989) 'Medical Paternalism: Blowing the Whistle'. *Solicitors Journal* 132; 25(9): 10–11.

Toeller, M. (1993) 'Diet in diabetes'. *Medicine International*. 21(7): 245–7.

Tomlinson, D.R. (1994) 'Aldose reductase: its importance in diabetes'. *Practical Diabetes*. 11(2): 51–4.

Townsend, P. and N. Davidson (eds) (1992) *Inequalities in Health: The Black Report and The Health Divide*. Penguin: London

Turner, R. (1993) 'Non-insulin dependent diabetes mellitus'. *Medicine International*. 21(7): 257–60.

UK Prospective Diabetes Study Group. (1998a) 'Intensive blood glucose control with sulphonylureas or insulin compared with conventional treatment and risk of complications in patients with type 2 diabetes: UKPDS 33'. *Lancet*. 352: 837–53.

UK Prospective Diabetes Study Group. (1998b) 'Tight blood pressure control and risk of macrovascular and microvascular complications in type 2 diabetes: UKPDS 38. *British Medical Journal*. 317: 703–11.

UK Prospective Diabetes Study Group. (1998c) 'Efficacy of atenolol and captopril in reducing macrovascular and microvascular complications in type 2 diabetes: UKPDS 39'. *British Medical Journal*. 317: 713–26.

UKCC (1992a) *Code of Professional Conduct*. UKCC: London.

UKCC (1992b) *Standards for the Administration of Medicines*. UKCC: London.

UKCC (1992c) *The Scope of Professional Practice*. UKCC: London.

UKCC (1994) *The future of Professional Practice Following Registration (PREP)*. UKCC: London.

UKCC (1996) *Guidelines for Professional Practice*. United Kingdom Central Council for Nursing, Midwifery and Health Visiting: London.

UKCC (1998) *Guidelines for Records and Record Keeping*. London: UKCC.

Unwin, N., S. Carr, J. Leeson and T. Pless-Mulloll (1997) *An introduction Study Guide to Public Health and Epidemiology*. Open University Press: Buckingham.

Van der Molen, T., D. S. Postma, M.O. Turner (1996) 'Effects of the long acting beta agonist formoterol on asthma control in asthmatic patients using inhaled steroids'. *Thorax*. 52: 535–9.

Vathenen, A.S., A.J. Knox, A. Wisniwski and A.E. Tattersfield (1991) 'Time course of change in bronchial reactivity with an inhaled corticosteroid in asthma'. *American Review of Respiratory Disease*. 142: 1317–21.

Wallace, H., S. Shorvon and A. Hopkins (eds) (1997) *Adults with Poorly Controlled Epilepsy: Clinical Guidelines for Treatment and Practical Tools for Aiding Epilepsy Management*. Royal College of Physicians: London.

Warner, J. (1991) 'The influence of exposure to house dust mite on sensitisation in asthma'. *Paediatric Allergy and Immunology*. 1: 79–86.

Warner, J.O. and J.F. Price (1978) 'House dust mite sensitivity in childhood asthma'. *Archives of Disease in Childhood*. 53: 710–13.

Watkins, P.J. (1993) 'Diagnosis and treatment of diabetic nephropathy'. *Medicine International*. 21(7): 264–5.

Whelton, P.K. (1994) 'Epidemiology of hypertension'. *Lancet*. 344: 101–6.

Whelton, P.K., J. He, J.A. Cutler, F.L. Brancati, L.J., Appel, D. Follmann and M.J. Klag (1997) 'Effects of oral potassium on blood pressure'. *Journal of the American Medical Association*. 277(20): 1624–32.

Whitehead, M. (1987) *The Health Divide*. Health Education Council: London.

Whitehead, M. (ed.) (1992) *Inequalities in Health*. Penguin: Harmondsworth.

WHO and IDF (1989) *The St Vincent Declaration*. WHO: Geneva.

Williams, E.I. (1993) *Health Checks for People Aged 75 and Over*. Royal College of General Practitioners Occasional Paper 59.

Wilson, J. and G. Junger (1968) *Principles and Practice of Screening for Disease*. Public Health Papers No. 34. WHO: Geneva.

Wise, E. (1986) 'The Social ulcer'. *Nursing Times*. May 21–27 82(21): 47–9.

Wolthers, O.D., S. Pederson (1993) 'Short term growth during treatment with inhaled fluticasone and becomethasone dipropionate'. *Archives Disease of Childhood*. 68: 673–76.

Woolcock, A., B. Lundback, N. Ringdal and L.A. Jacques (1996) 'Comparison of addition of salmeterol to inhaled steroids with doubling of the dose of inhaled steroids'. *Am J Respir Care Med*. 154: 141–8.

World Health Organisation (1978) Report on the International Conference on Primary Health Care, Alma Ata, 6–12 September. WHO: Copenhagen.

Wright, J. (1990) *Building and Using a Model of Nursing*. (2nd edn) Edward Arnold: London.

Young, A. and J. Tingle (1995) Record Keeping. *British Journal of Nursing*. 4(3): 179.

Young, A.P. (1994) 'In the Patients Best Interest. Law and Professional Conduct'. Chapter 9. In:

G. Hunt (ed.) *Ethical Issues in Nursing*. Routledge: London.

Zimmet, P. (1993) 'Diabetes: definitions and classification'. *Medicine International*. 21(7): 237–9.

Index